SURVIVE
and ADVANCE

My Cancer Battle,
Fought One Laugh at a Time

STEVE
ABBOTT

P
PRAUSPRESS

FIRST EDITION

Published by Praus Press
306 Greenup, Covington, KY 41011
www.prauspress.com

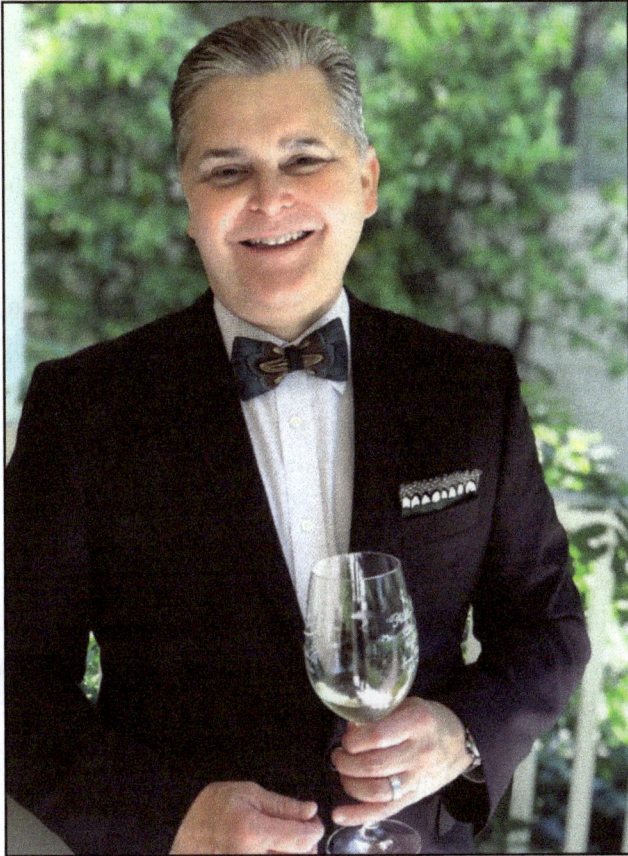

Steve at the Mondavi Family's 100th anniversary live auction.

INTRODUCTION

by Donna Salyers, founder of Fabulous Furs,
honored as a Great Living Cincinnatian

STEVE Abbott is an enigma — in the best possible way. I first met Steve when, as a volunteer for American Cancer Society (ACS), he stopped by Fabulous Furs to pick up our donation for the ACS Striders' Ball. With choirboy demeanor masking the stealth of a heat-seeking missile, Steve somehow recruited me to serve on the Striders' Ball Ambassador Board. I suspect every member of our Board had a similar story, and we all looked forward to the bi-weekly meetings which Steve made enjoyable and productive.

A solid "numbers guy," Steve likes to refer to himself as a "recovering accountant." When Monteverdi Tuscany, an upscale boutique resort based in Italy with a Cincinnati owner, needed a CFO to handle management, capital structure decisions, and risk management, plus banking and investor relationships, Steve was the man.

Steve's marketing skills soon thereafter came to the fore. As Monteverdi grew and expanded, he became the Chief Development Officer, adding responsibilities for generating new business opportunities and building strategic partnerships and collaborations in his role. In addition, he managed travel agent and tour operator relationships; created non-standard stay options; and served as Monteverdi's public face at industry and philanthropic events.

As everyone knows, Covid-19 closed tourism worldwide in 2020. Monteverdi's entire staff was let go. Steve became Executive Director of the Cincinnati Cancer Foundation and entered the nonprofit world. This once-shy accountant now wields a microphone once a week as the founder and host of the Cincinnati Cancer Advisors' 'Medical Minute' podcast.

But for you, dear reader, there's yet another area where Steve rises above the rest — he's also an excellent wordsmith. You're about to read an intimate account of the travails and triumphs of his own cancer treatment, the gained wisdom, and the ups and downs. Steve's prostate cancer diagnosis came in July 2013. It's estimated that nearly 300,000 cases of prostate cancer were diagnosed in the US in 2023, which makes it the most common cancer among men after skin cancer. Typically low risk, 97% of those diagnosed with prostate cancer survive 15 years after diagnosis.

But in Steve's case, despite immediate surgery, it's been anything but low risk. Following surgery nearly eleven years ago at this writing, Steve has remained in continuous treatment. He's experienced the prayerful anticipation of countless experimental drug trials...only to be followed by the crushing disappointment of dismal results. At his side through it all has been his lovely wife, Diana, a cancer survivor herself.

Few people can write about cancer with humor. Let alone "LOL" humor. Steve has managed to transform his cancer journey into an entertaining trip through pop culture. Using movie lines — "Hey brother, can you spare $66,515"— and song lyrics, — "Go back, Jack, do it again" — Steve writes with self-effacing wit. Not an easy task to address a subject as serious as cancer, especially his own. This is why I'm so pleased Steve is sharing his story with the world. His experiences will no doubt clear a path for countless cancer patients, and not just prostate cancer.

Recently, Steve received the "Caesar Blevins Warrior Award" from ZERO Prostate Cancer in Washington, D.C. He was also named an "Unsung Hero" by Cancer Family Care and "Nonprofit Executive Director of the Year" by Medical Mutual. In February 2024, Steve spoke on cancer survivorship to more than 1,000 pharmaceutical industry representatives in Orlando. It's been quite an upward journey due to his achievements, and downward as you will see, evolution from his wedding day when he nearly passed out from the stress of having to recite his wedding vows in front of 100 family members and friends. Steve credits cancer as being the driving force behind his impassioned mission to reduce the lethality of this hideous disease.

Just so you know, that guy in the oncology waiting room who's laughing like crazy? He's probably also reading Steve's book, the same one you have in your hands right now. Enjoy and prepare to be charmed by *Survive and Advance*.

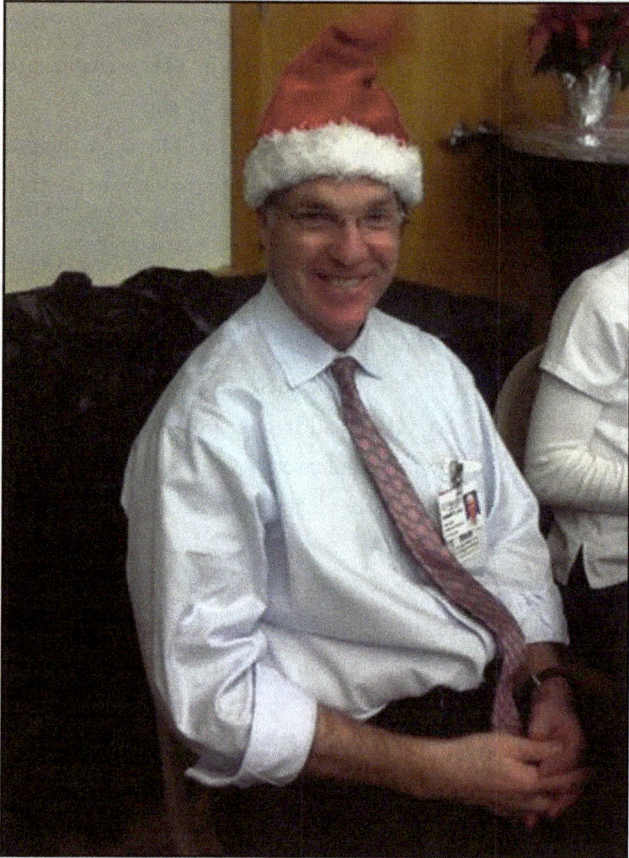

Dr. William L. "Bill" Barrett, founder and Chairman of the Board
of Cincinnati Cancer Foundation, Inc. Bill is also Co-Director and
Chairman of the Department of Radiation Oncology at the University
of Cincinnati Cancer Center.

PREFACE *and* DEDICATION

AUGUST 13, 2013. It was a Tuesday. In terms of world history, no treaties were signed and no weather disasters had folks sheltered in place. Notably in U.S. country music, Luke Bryan dropped his 4th studio record album. For local sports fans, the Cincinnati Reds beat the Chicago Cubs, 6-4.

But for myself, August 13, 2013, was the day that split my life in two, from, (1) a happy, workaday, successful, yet largely unremarkable track up until then, and (2) everything that would come thereafter.

Because August 13, 2013 was the day I received a prostate cancer diagnosis.

Just two months prior, my friend Rob Bolte passed away from lymphoma. A larger-than-life character who knew no strangers. For years, he had battled a variety of health issues, most of which appeared to be digestive in nature. There had been several diagnoses, or at least theories, along the way, including Celiac disease.

Following a family vacation to the Dominican Republic, Rob's condition suddenly worsened. Medical experts weighed in on what the problem might be. At one point, it was suspected that he might have even contracted Dengue Fever. By the time lymphoma was confirmed, Rob had only days to live.

Two nights before his passing, I stood in his hospital room, bewildered. My boisterous, gregarious, full-of-life friend was a shell of his former self: non-responsive, sustained only by being connected to a variety of machines. While I knew things were dire, I could not reconcile how he could be failing so quickly. Now that his team of hematologists knew definitively what the problem was, it still didn't mean that there was a playbook for treating this successfully.

I somehow expected a miracle.

The miracle never came.

Rob's passing was not only heartbreaking — it was also a shock to everyone. It's no stretch to say that no one in his circle of family or friends could believe it. In addition to the emotional pain we all felt, I thought "if someone like Rob could die at the age of 42, none of us are safe." At the risk of using a cliché, it was a personal wake-up call. I had been both busy and lazy with my own health care. To be clear, I was in good physical shape at the time. I had been working out, and for whatever reason, I was on a no-sugar kick. I had lost quite a bit of weight, even to the point of concern for some of my family. I was 5' 10" and weighed 135 pounds.

Because I had felt well, I hadn't made time for regular medical visits. In the wake of Rob's death, I scheduled a day off from work for overdue exams with my primary care physician, optometrist, and dentist.

My father had been diagnosed with prostate cancer when I was 44 years old. At that point, all I knew about prostate cancer was its proclivity to pass to other male family members. As such, I scheduled a urology visit with a randomly chosen urologist close to my home, figuring that I would likely need a relationship with a urologist sometime in the future. It was a fateful choice.

As luck would have it, the urologist was the first appointment on the calendar; Tuesday, July 2, 2013. Given my long tenure with the company I worked for at the time, I was flush with vacation time. Also on Tuesday, July 2, 2013, Rush, one of my favorite rock bands ever, was playing at Riverbend Music Center in Cincinnati that evening. My brother Brad and I bought great seats, an ideal kickoff to a long holiday weekend .

Due to an apparent lack of symptoms, I anticipated a quick visit to the urologist (the best kind of urology visit!).

It was anything but.

After an initial discussion of my medical history, the urologist moved swiftly to the dreaded "digital rectal exam". For most men, this is the annual nightmare that none of us want to think about. Enlightened men also know that women tolerate something equally bad, if not worse, on a yearly basis as well. They just complain about it less and do it more.

This exam hurt. My grimace was accompanied by his immediate observation that it should not have hurt that badly. He came right out with it: he felt a "large lump" that was consistent with prostate cancer. The "C" word. Cancer. He said that we needed to collect some blood to see what my PSA was, but he told me that he felt certain that prostate cancer would ultimately be confirmed.

My brother and I still went to the concert that evening. Despite my lifelong love of that band, and my knowledge of their entire songbook, I barely remember that show. I couldn't think of anything else while the show was going on except "oh my God, do I have cancer?" It was planned to be such a fun weekend — what in the world happened on the way to the show?

Back in the immediate aftermath of my father's diagnosis, I had previously had a PSA done. I was 44 at the time and my PSA was 0.4 ng/dl.. Golden. No problem. This time, my PSA came back at 10.8. Although somewhat arbitrary, prostate cancer is generally suspected when a man's PSA rises above 4.0 ng/dl. My urologist pulled no punches in telling me that a biopsy would be required to definitively diagnose the condition, but he repeated that he suspected prostate cancer.

By August 13, 2013, the empirical evidence proved conclusive: a large, palpable lump. Not only was my PSA high, my PSA "velocity" was also high, having risen from 0.4 to 10.8 in six years. The biopsy found prostate cancer cells in every "core" that was tested. Yet I felt fine and did not seem to have any of the symptoms. I could not believe it. My wife Diana and I traveled the state of Ohio for the next several weeks — to some excellent cancer centers in Columbus and Cleveland, all in search of someone to tell me that this diagnosis was incorrect. Everyone agreed with the initial diagnosis -I had prostate cancer.

I chose to have a radical prostatectomy as the first line of defense. Prior to my scheduled surgery with a renowned urologic surgeon in Columbus, he started our consultation with a sense of urgency my wife and I were not prepared for. He asked if we had any upcoming plans and I told him that we had a vacation scheduled over Labor Day. He asked if we'd be willing to cancel that vacation if he could juggle his surgical schedule in order to perform the surgery as soon as possible. He told us that he was optimistic, but even with the expedited surgery, he could not guarantee that he could "get it all" As it turns out, he was correct.

Roughly 70% of the men who are diagnosed with prostate cancer will choose a "first-line" therapy of surgery or radiation, which most often eradicates the cancer with no recurrence. Most in that group will live more than five years, no matter what course of treatment they choose.

It is now over a decade later and I am not cancer-free. I have never been able to enjoy hearing words like "you are cured" or "there is no evidence of disease" or "you are in remission."

My journey has been different. I have been in continuous treatment for advanced prostate cancer since Tuesday, September 3, 2013, when my prostate gland was removed.

The book you now hold in your hands has evolved from a largely lighthearted blog I began writing in February 2022 to chronicle my cancer treatment journey. My hope was that by sharing my experience, I'd be able to impart some wisdom, or at least experience, to prostate cancer patients, plus other cancer patients in general. I am not a medical professional so I took great pains to try not to overstep or dispense any medical advice. At every turn, I try to be a well-informed patient and I do try to help pass along my learnings in hopes that it might help guys to better understand their choices when facing these bewildering treatment options.

Along for the ride is whatever measure of wisdom that I may have gained from facing a life- threatening disease. To wit, I now know that I will not live as long as I would like to...but who ever does? As I write this in April 2024, there have been recent ominous developments in my case that are very concerning. I have cycled through almost every FDA-approved therapy yet my cancer has been resistant to those therapies. Clinical trials are still an option, but many of those are at an early stage with limited safety data. I personally know of people that have entered clinical trials only to pass away shortly thereafter.

None of this is lost on me.

One of the novelties of that original blog concept was that I tried to limit each entry to 500 words, for reasons that will be further explained later. As such, and ironically enough, this preface will likely end up being one of the longest "chapters" you will read. A new development — courtesy of my dear friend Donna Salyers and a well-known local book publisher (thank you, Richard) is that this blog has been recast, designed, printed and bound as this book. It has only been in recent days that I have come up with a title and subtitle for the book. I am not sure yet how I will fund it, but I will find a way. I intend for this project to be a charity fundraiser for Cincinnati Cancer Advisors, an organization that I'm proud to represent as its Executive Director. My goal is to leave something behind that might help a few more people in some meaningful way.

My original title for the blog when I began it in February 2022 was 5 Years; 500 Words at a Time, reflecting my goal of living five more years with advanced prostate cancer. Despite the comparatively favorable cancer journey of people with prostate cancer relative to other cancers, living 14 years with advanced prostate cancer would be a pretty good accomplishment. That is still my goal, but my brain (and recent test results) tells me I am not going to meet that goal. Publishing this (albeit short) book in mid-to-late 2024 reflects my desire to draft a finished manuscript while I am still doing relatively well as I still hope to steal victory from the jaws of defeat with the help of additional research discoveries and my own sheer determination.

The short chapters reflect my own undiagnosed attention-span disorder. My shelves are littered with half-read books. My intentions are always good when I start a book, but due to "squirrel" syndrome (if you know, you know), I rarely finish a 300-page book. This book will clock in at much less than that, i.e., one that even I can get through.

This book is the result of the encouragement of many people, but it is ultimately dedicated to Rob Bolte. I am alive today because of the timing of his passing, which was unconscionable at his young age. He left his family and many friends behind. His passing can never be redeemed, but there was at least one good outcome from it. I hope I can do the same for someone else. Thank you for reading my book.

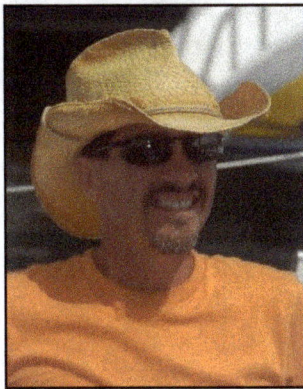

My friend Rob Bolte, who lost his battle with lymphoma way too soon at age 42.

FIVE YEARS;
500 WORDS AT A TIME

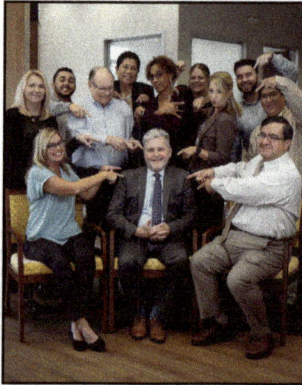

My friends/colleagues/Cincinnati Cancer Advisors family members, left to right (with me in the center): Sally Hellard, Diana Abbott, Jake DeHart, Phil Leming, Aoy Sefchik, Sherry Hughes, Christine Desso, Jill Hunt, Chris McNeil, Andy Guinigundo and Abdul Jazieh.

FEBRUARY 15, 2022 - For anyone who does not know me, I serve as the Executive Director of the Cincinnati Cancer Foundation, which is the PERFECT job for me at this stage of my life and career. Why? As a prostate cancer survivor, I represent an organization that — as stated by our founder Dr. Bill Barrett - exists to (a) reduce the suffering and mortality that often accompanies a cancer diagnosis and (b) make Cincinnati, Ohio the best city in the country to live in if one must face this formidable mortal adversary.

This book came to life for multiple reasons. First, my wife, Diana, has been telling me for years that I should "become a writer." Diving into an already crowded pool seemed beyond me, and since I prefer not to starve, I have never pursued "authorship" in any meaningful way.

But the second reason — my wanting to empower fellow cancer survivors to make better and more informed decisions about their oncology care — eventually overrode my hesitancy.

Last, my cancer has now metastasized to distant sites — most recently my left lung, neck, and liver. These are ominous developments that threaten my long-term survival.

I decided to title my blog *5 Years; 500 Words at a Time* because only 30% of prostate cancer patients who have become resistant to hormone therapy are expected to live for five years. My original intention was to live at least five more years; a goal I still cling to despite the recent stop sticks thrown into my path by cancer.

The next phase of my treatment journey will go right to the heart of what we exist to do here at Cincinnati Cancer Advisors which is to improve the outcomes of cancer patients through better, more involved, passionate health care using "all resources that exist on Planet Earth to help in all ways that we can to improve patients' diagnoses and their care by giving them hope they're not without the potential of a better day tomorrow" (I stole this quote from our Medical Director, Dr. Phil Leming).

I hoped to use the online forum to educate patients and keep the many wonderful people in my life who care about me updated on my cancer journey. My cancer is progressing, and my understanding is whatever we do next from a treatment perspective needs to kick off soon.

In the meantime, I am starting to plan for what I need to get done over the next four to six months during a time when I might not be feeling so well, or at full strength.

TOM PETTY WAS
ON TO SOMETHING

ONE of my favorite Tom Petty songs is "The Waiting." I remember listening to it on the iconic Cincinnati radio station WEBN all the way back in 1981.

My job title back then was a lowly "Sign Printer" at Value City Department Store in Latonia, Kentucky. I had a ramshackle "office" (more like a cage over the loading dock — think Louie from the TV show "Taxi" but with no authority) that always smelled of diesel fuel from the delivery trucks and ink and solvent from my primitive print shop. The silver lining was that I was one of the very few employees in the store allowed to listen to the radio during the day. Given my lifelong love of music, it was a nice trade-off for getting my hands dirty, something that still, by my own admission, I am loath to do even at this stage of my life.

So how does a Tom Petty song become part of a soundtrack in a cancer journey? One thing that cancer survivors learn fast is that sometimes, the waiting is the hardest part. It begins before you are even officially classified as a cancer patient or survivor. Waiting days for a biopsy result that you simultaneously want and dread at the same time. For many cancer survivors, that fearful waiting feeling continues every three, six or twelve months while anticipating test results, hoping against hope that there has been no recurrence or disease progression in the meantime.

I remember the nervous waiting that Diana and I shared after my first post-prostatectomy PSA like it was yesterday (PSA is a protein that appears on cells in the prostate gland that can be indicative of a variety of conditions, including prostate cancer). In order to be cured, my PSA needed to be somewhere down around 0.01...but mine was 0.10. My urologist suggested that we do another blood draw in a month, hoping that there might be some lingering cancer cells that would be gone by then. The result was 0.2. I was not cured by the surgery. I began salvage radiation treatment in January 2014. The thinking was the cancer was still localized so radiation would obliterate the rest of it.

Thirty-three radiation treatments later, my PSA has never come down.

My cancer is incurable (but treatable).

That reality kicked off a cycle of waiting for test results every three months. In the beginning, I would literally pull over to the side of the road whenever I got a push notification on my phone alerting me that the most recent test result had been posted to my patient portal. I couldn't wait until

I got home for the news. I am sure I'm not the only cancer patient that has experienced this anxiety.

My brother Brad has reminded me of another great Tom Petty lyric: "most things I worry about never happen anyway." Cancer patients must get really good at taking a deep breath, not assuming the worst, and not going down the Google rabbit hole in researching their disease and prognosis.

It's harder than it sounds sometimes.

THE MEDIAN IS NOT THE MESSAGE

STEVE ABBOTT

THIS post is dedicated to my friend Brian Gillan, whose wife Paula is a breast cancer survivor, also a friend, and a great supporter of Cincinnati Cancer Advisors.

I distinctly remember the panic I felt when I first learned I had prostate cancer. Three separate medical opinions provided uniform consensus that I needed to act quickly, whereas acting quickly is often not required with prostate cancer. The interval between my diagnosis and the first operation was necessarily short.

I had plenty of time off work after my prostatectomy. Maybe too much time. So much time that I descended into a dark place trying to determine my prognosis. I assumed the worst, which at that time was much more in line with my personality than it is now. Assuming the worst is a means of self-protection. For if the news was better than feared, then great. Time to celebrate! But if the news was as bad as assumed, well, I was no worse off.

I can't imagine living that way now.

The main reason why I can't imagine living that way now is because of an essay, written by Stephen Jay Gould, an American paleontologist, biologist and scientist, that my friend Brian Gillan sent me after one of our heart-to-heart conversations about life. The essay was entitled "The Median Is Not the Message."

See, Gould was diagnosed with peritoneal mesothelioma in 1982, a deadly form of cancer that targets the abdominal lining. Gould's background in research put him in a good position to logically deconstruct what he was reading in medical literature. The literature at the time stated that Gould's disease was incurable, with a "median mortality" of eight months after discovery.

Gould noted that the median is not the average (as many people assume). Instead, the median is the halfway point. Statistically, that means that 50% of the people with his diagnosis would die within eight months and 50% would die more than eight months later. Gould was 40 years old at the time and otherwise in good health. He reasoned that the 50% who died in eight months or less were more likely to have been elderly with significant comorbidities and/or other risk factors which did not apply in his case. Basically, he concluded that the median statistic was meaningless to his case… i.e., it did not apply to his cancer.

Understanding his logic has allowed me to view these types of statistics with a baseball-size grain of salt. That said, I do use these often-gloomy predictions as fuel to live my life with urgency, passion, and gratitude. Gould died 20 years, not 20 months, later from a completely unrelated lung cancer. I have shared his essay with many other frightened patients and I hope it helped them too. Thanks for the share, Brian!

HEY BROTHER,
CAN YOU SPARE $66,515?

ONE of the good things about staying as busy as I have been lately is that I haven't had time to check in on my mounting medical bills. Finally, though, curiosity got the better of me so I logged into my various patient portals.

Just for fun, I added everything up since December 17, 2022 — the date when my latest PSA result took off like a rocket ship — and this is what I found:

Total amounts billed = $67,686, less insurance payments = ($1,171) ... amount I owe: $66,515

I am not panicking because, unfortunately, I have been down this road a few times before. That said, I can confidently predict three things: (1) a decent chunk of the amount owed will end up being paid by my insurance company; (2) a decent chunk of it won't end up being paid by my insurance company, and; (3) it's going to chew up a decent chunk of my time to sort it all out. This calculation does not even include charges for the genetic profiling that has been sent to Caris Life Sciences on the enlarged lymph nodes in my neck.

Strangely enough, I worry more about other people who end up in this situation, more than I do myself. Although far from being young, I am at least young enough to be reasonably tech savvy so I can keep track of where I am in the process. I am very accustomed to advocating for myself after nearly a decade of continuous cancer treatment. I am blessed to have a good education and a good job, plus savings to lean on.

But what if all these things weren't the case? If not, I might end up holding the bag for thousands (or even tens of thousands) of dollars.

These types of experiences are why I am so passionate about patient financial navigation services. It's why I pursued a partnership between Cincinnati Cancer Advisors (CCA) and the Patient Advocate Foundation (PAF) in the summer of 2021. By partnering with PAF, we can help our patients resolve these types of issues, as well as get enrolled for medical insurance plans they don't yet have, and even access forms of public assistance that will help keep their utilities from being turned off or being evicted from their home while they struggle to resolve these issues.

Partly due to this partnership between CCA and PAF, CCA representatives met with City of Cincinnati Mayor Aftab Pureval to present our "Gift to the City." CCA is now offering to help patients not just with cancer, but with other forms of chronic, debilitating, and life-threatening diseases. Although it is an overused cliché, we really are all in this together.

I hope that more patients take us up on our offer — the last thing people need when they are not at their best is having to battle huge corporations to get their bills covered.

GO BACK, JACK, DO IT AGAIN

ONE maddening thing that people who have worked closely with me know is that I believe that pretty much everything that happens in life can be tied to one of three things:

1. A line from a movie.
2. A scene from a "Seinfeld" episode.
3. A song lyric.

While driving back from Morgantown, WV yesterday, I fiddled nonstop with the Sirius XM stations (as I always do), looking for the perfect song. Somehow, I ended up on the "Classic Rewind" station where I hung out for a few songs. Steely Dan's *"Do It Again"* came on, and even though I was never much of a Steely Dan fan, I left it on because — let's face it — it's still a pretty cool song.

Once the chorus started, I laughed because I had been thinking about the events of the last week. You see, I had a biopsy of three lymph nodes in my neck where cancer had been found lurking. This location (i.e., the neck) is not consistent with prostate cancer, but it's also not out of the realm of reason that it could have spread there.

Part of the tissue from that biopsy was sent off to Caris Life Sciences, "Caris" a really important step.

Why, you ask? Thanks to advances in genetic profiling and molecular medicine, you can now create a genetic profile of a person's individual cancer. That information, combined with years of research data, can lead to very specific treatment protocols that can improve the outcomes for cancer patients. This information can lead to two very specific improvements in treatment: (1) it can help to avoid treatments that won't work and (2) steer the patient's oncology team to treatments that might work better.

After 16 days, I received my report and quickly scanned the multi-page report and nearly everywhere I looked, I saw "QNS." Even with my limited layman's understanding, I knew this didn't sound right. In looking at the legend for the report, I learned that QNS means "quantity not sufficient." There was not enough tissue sent to Caris for them to determine whether I was BRCA 1 or BRCA 2 positive, which is a cornerstone piece of information for formulating my treatment plan. UGH. Thankfully, the hospital's surgical pathology lab had more tissue in their "tissue bank," which they sent to Caris. But in the meantime, we are starting all over again.

If I am BRCA 1 or BRCA 2 positive (about a 15% to 20% chance), I will likely go on the least invasive form of treatment called a "PARP inhibitor." If not, we will consider a range of clinical trials that would likely combine a proven drug with immunotherapy (i.e. Keytruda - a "checkpoint inhibitor") and another investigational drug not yet FDA approved. Chemotherapy is still an option, but it is the least preferred option at this point.

Indeed, sometimes the waiting is the hardest part.

CHECK MY BRAIN

TODAY was a "rule-out" type of test, specifically "let's make sure the cancer has not metastasized to your brain." Although unlikely to find it there, it was a necessary step since the prostate cancer was found in a place it does not normally go — my neck — which was not that far from my brain.

I am happy to report two outcomes from today's test result:

1. They actually found a brain in there.

2. They did not find any trace of cancer in my brain (so that is pretty cool).

One funny thing though. The radiation tech (Sarah) asked me what Pandora station I wanted to listen to during the 30 minutes I had to stay motionless in the MRI machine. With a brain MRI, you want to make sure to choose something good, otherwise it sounds like a jackhammer going off in the headphones. I told her Linkin Park and she said, "great choice." Once I got in the tube, I heard nothing but "yacht rock" selections like Toto's "Africa," Christopher Cross' "Sailing" and Norm Greenbaum's "Spirit in the Sky." Seriously? The only conclusion I could draw was that the Linkin Park Pandora channel was considered incompatible in cases where brain health and brain activity are being assessed.

As I quietly stayed motionless in the tube — suffering through yacht rock — the perfect song lyric popped into my head... "somebody check my brain." The song "Check My Brain" is hands-down one of my favorite Alice in Chains songs. I still can't get enough of it. Although it is just one step along the way, I am glad that someone checked my brain today, and it was fine (i.e. no cancer).

Tomorrow, I will meet with my medical oncologist. Hopefully, I will move one step closer to figuring out what my treatment plan looks like.

In the meantime, I think I will fire up a bit of Alice in Chains before going to bed.

If I am BRCA 1 or BRCA 2 positive (about a 15% to 20% chance), I will likely go on the least invasive form of treatment called a "PARP inhibitor." If not, we will consider a range of clinical trials that would likely combine a proven drug with immunotherapy (i.e. Keytruda — a "checkpoint inhibitor") and another investigational drug not yet FDA approved. Chemotherapy is still an option, but it is the least preferred option at this point.

Indeed, sometimes the waiting is the hardest part.

STEVE ABBOTT

A HOBSON'S CHOICE

THE Merriam-Webster dictionary defines a "Hobson's Choice" as "an apparently free choice when there is no real alternative." That's a pretty good description of where I find myself right now.

Following surgery to remove my cancerous prostate gland in 2013 and salvage radiation in early 2014 to hopefully eradicate any remaining prostate cancer cells, I began a new treatment phase in 2017 thatis often referred to as "hormone therapy". With ADT, prostate cancer cells are deprived of testosterone — a fuel that helps them to thrive and proliferate — with pernicious effects on a man's lifestyle and quality of life. Whereas normal levels of testosterone are about 300 — 1,000 nanograms per deciliter in a man's blood, mine has vacillated between 3ng/dl to 25 ng/dl for the last five years. Given that a prostate cancer cell's uptake of testosterone is akin to me drinking wine on a trip to Napa Valley, I have been very grateful to be on this class of drugs that has clamped down on my cancer for the last 5+ years.

One of my favorite Led Zeppelin songs is "When the Levee Breaks." A famous line from that song is "when the levee breaks, I'll have no place to stay." That's where I find myself now as I can no longer stay where I am at, nor where I have been. Prostate cancer has found a new pathway and is no longer responding to ADT, so I need to do something different.

My medical oncologist informed me that the next phase of my treatment will be something of a paradox. When discussing a clinical trial that may involve a chemotherapy drug, he said that one of the "uncomfortable and counterintuitive things about your upcoming treatment is that while you feel well now, I have to make you feel sick so that you will feel better later." So, it's a classic Hobson's Choice wherein you are choosing to do something you don't have to do, but yet there is no real alternative.

The levee has indeed broken on ADT, so doing nothing is neither a practical nor wise option. Thankfully, I don't have other comorbidities such as diabetes, heart disease, circulatory system issues, so I am in a good position to take this on. Nonetheless, it is slightly terrifying to read the "informed consent" documents that I need to sign to be accepted into the clinical trial that's been recommended for me.

It's damn daunting to willingly enter a clinical trial that relies on a handful of unproven, non-FDA approved drugs. Yet it would be disingenuous of me to stand on the shoulders of people that have gone through previous clinical trials and not be willing to do it myself. Their willingness to participate has resulted in the FDA-approved drugs that have kept me alive and well for nearly a decade at this point.

Therefore, I am thinking of it in terms of fixing your roof or waterproofing your basement before the heavens open up and you are trying to mop away water (or rogue cells) from places they were never meant to be.

NEW NEWS = NO NEWS

WELL, I have news to share, but it feels that not much has changed. The second report from Caris was helpful, but it certainly didn't provide any crystal-clear next steps.

There was an unequivocal finding that I am negative for a BRCA-1 or BRCA-2 genetic mutation, which rules out the use of a newer drug showing good efficacy with prostate cancer called Olaparib (aka Lynparza). In the plus column, though, is that I *think* the negative BRCA results bode well for my two sisters not developing breast cancer in the future.

But the report did show that I am positive for an AR V7 variant, which indicates that the prostate cancer is now becoming resistant to anti-androgen therapy (which we kind of already knew based on my quickly rising PSA and where the cancer was recently found).

Outside of that, the report did not show an "actionable target," which in layman's terms, pretty much means I just must make a decision and roll with it.

As I type this, I am waiting for an updated PSA result. I started a new androgen blockade drug called Casodex a few weeks ago which is strictly a bridge medication to try to control things a bit until we know what the next steps are. Casodex is one of the very oldest of the anti-androgen drugs so I am not expecting to see much cancer control out of it; we shall see.

I have a choice of two clinical trials — one at the National Institutes of Health in Bethesda, Maryland, the other at the University of Michigan in Ann Arbor. My medical oncologist agrees with my preference for the trial in Ann Arbor which relies more on a combination of FDA-approved drugs rather than none of the drugs being FDA-approved (i.e., the NIH in Bethesda). He also feels that I need to start on one of the two clinical trials or start chemotherapy within the next month.

Since it is likely — but by no means guaranteed — that I will get into one of the two clinical trials, my medical oncologist scheduled me to begin chemotherapy about a month from today. If I go the chemo route — in what can only be described as an incredible irony proving that the universe has a sense of humor — I will lose my hair. This would be a problem on two fronts: (1) my vanity when it comes to my hair and (2) my wife Diana is not a fan of guys wearing ball caps in the house.

FYI — I do have a lot of great ball caps thanks to our extensive travels, and I will not want to walk around bald, so we may have to have some sort of negotiated settlement over that one.

HOUSTON, WE HAVE A PROBLEM

ONE of the great benefits — and curses — of dealing with cancer over a long period of time is that you learn a lot more about cancer than you ever wanted to know...but not enough to really know what to do next. In a weird sort of way, choosing what to do next was probably easier in an era where there was less hope, and less information by way of treatment options.

Although I lived through that era of "less is more", I was too young to know what choices patients had to make. I suspect that their treatment choices were quite a bit more binary at that time since there were fewer treatments to choose from, and quite frankly, fewer doctors so there was not the same degree of subspeciality that there is now.

I am so fortunate to have a whole team of doctors looking out for me. Not only do I have an oncologist who has successfully managed my case for almost a decade at this point, but I also have a full team of oncologists at my workplace watching over me. Having five uber-qualified doctors is an incredible luxury that I do not take for granted, a luxury that I appreciate beyond words.

But that can also make things tricky though. I now have five clinicians with 100+ years of combined oncology experience reviewing every one of my test results. Everyone seems to agree that we are in an important place in time, i.e., where my cancer is spreading but I am still not symptomatic. They all seem to agree that a treatment decision needs to be made and started soon.

However, there is not widespread agreement on what that treatment choice should be.

Meanwhile, I find myself in the somewhat confusing position of having tremendous respect for each of these brilliant doctors, not being sure of what to do next, and not wanting to offend anyone by not following their advice. I guess you could say it is the downside of having an "embarrassment of riches" when it comes to medical advice.

One member of my oncology team asked me to visit MD Anderson Cancer Center in Houston, TX ("MD Anderson") to get the opinion of yet another oncologist there who deals almost exclusively with "genitourinary" cancers (FYI — genitourinary cancers are what I jokingly refer to as the "below the belt" cancers). Said another way, cancers of the body parts you don't really like to talk about in mixed company, if at all.

So I am checking into MD Anderson. This oncologist there is incredibly qualified; likewise, by most people's estimation, MD Anderson is one of the best cancer centers of excellence in the world. It takes a lot more paperwork to get accepted, but who wants to feel like they left anything on the table if they have an option?

Hopefully, Houston can help with this problem. Please accept my apologies for using such a cliched chapter title; it was right there and I had to grab it.

ONE STEP CLOSER TO THE EDGE

ONE of the many privileges extended to me over the years was an invitation to participate as one of only a few "consumer advocates" on a research panel for the Prostate Cancer Research Program. I was nominated by the former CEO of ZERO Prostate Cancer — Jamie Bearse — and I wanted to do it because it involved reviewing research proposals from scientists around the world who are trying to develop novel therapies and new approaches for dealing with advanced prostate cancer.

This program — which is ultimately managed by the U.S. Department of Defense (surprised? I was) — has funded research in the last decade alone that produced five groundbreaking drugs to combat advanced prostate cancer. I have been on several of these drugs, and they have no doubt extended my life by at least five years so far.

Trying to understand the "lay abstracts" that I had to review is on a par with trying to understand cryptocurrency and "blockchain" technology (which I do not understand and likely never will). It was great practice for reviewing "informed consents" for clinical trials that are laced with medical jargon, which I am doing now prior to making a very important treatment decision. But back to the clinical trial decision.

My interview with the National Institutes of Health resulted in acceptance into their trial, if that is what I want to do. However, on my newly developed Guinea Pig Scale, I would have to give this one four out of a possible five guinea pigs. I like that the trial is being run by the NIH and I like that it is free to patients. However, I'm not a huge fan of the fact that it relies entirely (like as in 100%) on "investigational" (i.e., unproven, non-FDA approved) drugs. The other thing is, although I used to spend huge amounts of time on airplanes, I am in no hurry to start traveling back-and-forth in a flying Petri dish, anticipating the side effects of four unapproved drugs being used in a novel combination for the first time in human beings. Yikes!

I also had a call with the Principal Investigator at the University of Michigan's Rogel Cancer Center last week to discuss a clinical trial they are offering which combines an immunotherapy drug (i.e., Keytruda — you've seen the commercials by now), a hormone therapy drug called Enzalutamide (that I have already been on and failed), and something called a "bromodomain inhibitor," which is designed to reduce the resistance to hormone therapy that I have developed and which unfortunately, allows my cancer to spread. I give this one only two guineas on the Guinea Pig Scale. If this trial is successful, hormone therapy drugs may begin to work again for some period of time, which would be awesome.

Thank God there are people out there who dedicate their lives to this research work, because I am not smart enough to do it myself. Looks like I might want to also begin researching the best wine bars, bottle shops, coffee emporiums and Mexican restaurants in Ann Arbor.

WHEN YOU COME TO A FORK IN THE ROAD, TAKE IT

I'M not sure who has coined the best quotes ever - Mark Twain, Winston Churchill, or Yogi Berra — but if you base it on sheer accidental brilliance, I say you have to go with Yogi's *"when you come to a fork in the road, take it."*

Many twists and turns have accompanied this attempt to get some clarity around what is going on with my disease and how to best deal with it. It has been a rocky road at times, especially since there was no real consensus among the many brilliant doctors who I spoke with about what the next step should be. Although there was no agreement as to the specific next steps, there was unanimous agreement that I had to do something.

This came when I went to get my quarterly Eligard injection. Eligard, like Lupron, is a drug that basically tricks the body to stop producing testosterone, which fuels prostate cancer cells to flourish. Eligard can only be injected directly into the stomach, which is not nearly as hilarious as the Lupron injections I get in my rear end. #humility

The appointment for the Eligard injection is always accompanied by extensive blood work, as organ toxicity can develop from long-term use of some of the hormone therapy drugs that I have been on over these many years. Despite being on these drugs for six years now, every... single... one... of the 42 different values in the hepatic function panel (liver values), renal function panel (kidney values), differential (% of white blood cells) and CBC (pretty much everything else) were perfect, except for the testosterone, which was a comically low 24 ng/dl on a normal scale of up to 1,000 ng/dl.

Then came the long wait for the PSA result. I was in a meeting with my oncologist when the result came back almost two hours later, and we did a high five when we saw that my PSA had DROPPED (from 21.9 to 15.8) for the first time in recent memory. I was shocked since I have only been on this new (but old) drug of Casodex for a month, so nobody really expected it to be very effective.

So, whereas consensus was previously hard to come by, all my docs now agreed that this PSA drop is a fork in the road, so I'm going to take it. No clinical trials at this time, and I'll stay on this drug until it looks like it is no longer working, then we'll figure out what to do next.

Cancer reminds you of your own fleeting existence and all this talk about cancer reminds me of another one of my favorite Yogi Berra quotes... *"you should always go to other people's funerals, otherwise, they won't come to yours."* Good words to live by!

HOTEL CALIFORNIA

IT feels good to be writing again after a two-week hiatus.

One of the best things about being married to your best friend of 40+ years is that your arguments can be restricted to the important stuff, like whether "Hotel California" is one of the best rock songs of all time. I am firmly on Team Hotel California, whereas Diana can't reach quickly enough to turn it off. She feels the same way about Don McLean's "American Pie" and Lynyrd Skynyrd's "Free Bird" so she appears to not like iconic seven-minute long rock anthems).

To say that I understand more than half of the lyrics to that song would be a stretch, but the one line I have always thought was brilliant that lends itself to so many situations is the chorus. *"Welcome to the Hotel California... you can check out, but you can never leave."* My journey with advanced prostate cancer has been very much like Hotel California.

Here are a few perceptions about prostate cancer that are generally true:
1. It is an "old man's" disease.
2. It is a slow-growing cancer.
3. You don't die of prostate cancer; you die with it.
Unless that is not the case...

My journey with prostate cancer has been vastly different than the 70+% of guys that are cured with no recurrence. Although I hope I die *with* prostate cancer and not of it, I recognize and accept that dying from prostate cancer is a possibility for me. A prime example was when I got the news that my PSA had decreased significantly in response to starting on a different drug.

But on the heels of this great news, I tried to check out of Hotel California. But before the valet could even bring my car around, my PSA started going back up again. With advanced prostate cancer, you can check out, but you can never leave.

Which brings me to my latest bit of "oncotourism," which was my trip to meet with a top specialist at MD Anderson that specializes in genitourinary cancers, and prostate cancer in particular. We reviewed a whole host of options yesterday afternoon, and my best option appears to be a clinical trial at MD Anderson that leverages the research findings behind the recently FDA- approved treatment of Pluvicto. The approval of Pluvicto has been eagerly anticipated by guys with advanced prostate cancer who are failing hormone therapy and need a way to either slow or reverse the growth of their prostate cancer.

Basically, the concept here is that the same "radiopharmaceutical" that is used to find prostate cancer cells lurking in the body in a PSMA PET scan can be armed with targeted radiation that can simultaneously begin killing those rogue cells. Pluvicto is currently only available to guys who have also had chemotherapy, but this clinical trial is for those that are failing hormone therapy but have not yet had chemo. I hope to find out soon whether I will be accepted into the trial. My goal today is the same as it was the day I was diagnosed... to die WITH prostate cancer and not OF it.

DENIAL IS NOT JUST
A RIVER IN EGYPT

MOST of us have heard that old line plenty of times, often attributed to Mark Twain. Whether you think it's corny or not, it's so brilliantly succinct and applies to so many situations in life that I am stealing it for today's chapter title. It also bring back a fun memory of seeing a street musician I only remember as "Jeff" who played 1970's hippie music in Charleston, SC standing next to a white bucket with a sign stating "Tipping is NOT a city in China."

We've also all heard the adage about insurance companies... that their strategy is "deny, deny, deny." Some assessments are less generous than that, referring to the "three D's of the insurance industry" as "delay, deny and defend."

I've mentioned this many times before, but perhaps the dirtiest little secret behind cancer treatment is the pernicious financial effects on patients that come from treating the disease that is trying to kill them. I spent this past weekend sorting through a huge database of medical claims data that I downloaded from my insurer. From this, I was able to ascertain that the remaining balance owed to my health care providers — in the absence of any further processing and after the insurance company has processed claims and made payments — is $99,120.85. Dollars, not pesos.

We filmed a video explaining how we got here, and hope to do additional videos as I work my way through this process. I am an unabashed fiscal conservative and social liberal, so I operate under the (faulty) premise that insurance companies have a right to make a buck, but I also believe they should do the right thing with the money they earn, beyond just taking care of their shareholders. In my mind, they also have a fiduciary duty to return value to subscribers in exchange for the premium payments they willingly accept. You can't fulfill that duty through a blanket denial of medical claims, ESPECIALLY when the claims you are denying are for people battling cancer.

The thing that frightens me is mustering the wherewithal to figure this stuff out. For better or for worse, I have spent my career managing databases and building financial models. As such, data doesn't scare me (and as my colleagues would tell you, I pretty much believe that anything worth doing is worth doing in Microsoft Excel).

But what about folks who can't sort this stuff out on their own? How do they even figure out what they really owe and how do they get help if their finances are crushed by the cost of treatment?

My experience underscores the reason why Cincinnati Cancer Advisors offers financial navigation services, and why we will have a continual focus on helping patients with financial navigation services. I don't know how to measure the negative effect on physical health that occurs when a patient is dealing with the new, crushing reality of insurmountable medical debt, but I know that it doesn't help. After nearly a decade of dealing with this stuff, I have learned how to roll with the punches, but I worry about those that are new to this game.

RUNNING TO STAND STILL

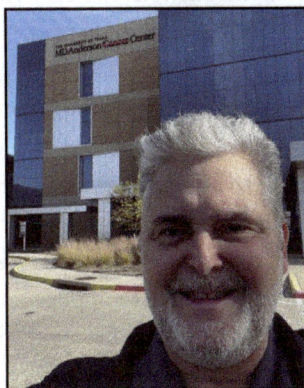

Me, arriving for my appointment with Dr. Christopher Logothetis at
MD Anderson Cancer Center in League City, Texas.

I feel like I have been "running to stand still" (one of my favorite U2 songs from the *"Joshua Tree"* album) for the last month.

An aim of both our *"Medical Minute"* video podcast series and this book is to give cancer patients insight into what cancer patients go through as part of their journey. My goal as Executive Director is not to complain about my cancer journey, but rather to educate and let patients know when and where Cincinnati Cancer Advisors can help.

Keeping this in mind, one thing I have tried to do is to convey the financial toxicity that can often accompany a cancer diagnosis. Lemme tell ya... neither the treatment nor the billing is for the faint of heart. I have recently learned the importance of "coordination of benefits" in the insurance billing setting, which becomes an issue if you have more than one medical plan. The confusion around that is what scored me aforementioned $99K in medical debt, which I am slowly working through.

The other part I wanted to update everyone on is the clinical trial option that I am pursuing at MD Anderson. After researching a variety of clinical trial options at different hospitals throughout the eastern U.S., my conclusion (as well as that of several members of my oncology team) was that the "PSMAfore" trial at MD Anderson was my best option.

The nice thing about this trial is that it is based on the same treatment protocol as what led to the FDA's recent approval of Pluvicto for advanced prostate cancer. This is a "radioligand" treatment that uses a PSMA PET scan (of which I have now had many) to not only find prostate cancer cells but concurrently deliver a potent dose of radiation that is designed to kill the cancer cells. That said, the recent FDA approval of Pluvicto applies only to guys whose PSA is progressing despite hormone therapy and have already had chemotherapy. By contrast, the PSMAfore trial does not require you to have previously had chemo, which is great for guys like me.

There's only one problem with that though, and it's a pretty big one. Novartis, the drug manufacturer, just voluntarily suspended production of the Lu 177 radio tracer that the clinical trial relies on, which means the clinical trial is on hold until further notice. Meanwhile, I just had an FDG PET scan a few weeks ago as a condition of getting into the trial but now I need to acquire a physical CD of the scan and upload it to MD Anderson. Two problems with that; (1) being provided with a copy of the scan on a CD and (2) finding a computer that even has a CD drive.

So, in summary, I am running hard, but currently just running to stand still.

ONE THING AFTER THE OTHER

THREE weeks ago, I recently experienced pain in my lower back. It seemed logical because we had just driven home from Hilton Head Island (about an 11-hour drive), so I initially chalked it up to lower back fatigue from making a long drive. The pain would ebb and flow from having bad pain for a day or maybe two, but then it would improve. So, each time, I felt like I might be turning the corner and didn't pursue treatment.

Four days ago, the pain became unbearable and included my right-side abdomen. I thought maybe things would improve again but I also knew that the pain level was so different that it warranted getting checked out. By last week, I couldn't take the pain anymore so Diana took me to urgent care (by this time, I could not stand up, bend over, or breathe without a significant amount of pain).

After a fairly worthless urgent care visit, it was decided that maybe I had a kidney stone that was blocked from passing, despite the fact that I tested negative for any blood in my urine. Urgent care prescribed two ineffective drugs that we picked up at the pharmacy. Upon arriving at home, I went directly to bed, hoping to find a position where I could get relatively comfortable (I couldn't).

After talking to my medical oncologist, and my friend/oncologist/mentor Dr. Bill Barrett, we decided it was prudent to get a CT scan of my abdomen to see whether the kidney stone could be seen on imaging. A few small kidney stones were seen, but none were of a size that would explain the pain increase. However, what did show up was an enlarged lymph node that had increased in size by almost 50%, and a cluster of newly enlarged lymph nodes.

The presumption is that the lymph nodes, enlarged due to cancer, are pressing on my ureter, and mimicking the symptoms of a "stuck" kidney stone. Meanwhile, this all has the potential to complicate the timing of getting into the clinical trial at MD Anderson, which will likely be a much more effective long-term strategy than stopgap measures.

One thing after another for sure, but to end this on a positive note, THANK GOD for Oxycodone. Stealing a line from one of my favorite Robert Plant songs, *I can breathe again!*

P.S. to Kevin Mooney — thanks for the pep talks. Even I need one of those occasionally.

WHINE COUNTRY

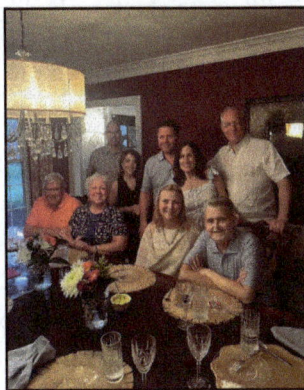

"Team Gerry" Front row, left to right: Chris Chalifoux, Nancy Chalifoux, Diana Abbott,
Steve Abbott. Back row, left to right: Sean Trivedi, Michele Trivedi, Joe Feldkamp,
Amy Feldkamp and Gerry Bollman.

OK, I'm going to do my best to not whine about the fact that I was supposed to spend this week in the Napa Valley drinking wine with some of my dearest friends. Unfortunately, cancer had a different set of plans for me.

Two additional cancerous spots have been located with a CT scan, but I was simultaneously celebrating the fact that Oxycodone (aka Percocet) had virtually eliminated all pain that I was experiencing from the cancerous lymph nodes pressing on my ureter.

Unless you have a reason to know this, you probably don't know it... but one of the downsides of using a narcotic to blunt pain is that it has the potential to create constipation. I began to experience that in a pretty severe way by about day three of taking the Oxycodone, so I promptly stopped taking it and figured I would just gut it out. Only one problem, by several days later with taking no Oxycodone, things were no better. In fact, they were much worse.

My radiation oncologist — believing that this did not sound right — went back and reviewed my recent scans with a radiologist and discovered that prostate cancer tumors had invaded my rectal wall, which is shrinking the size of that "passageway" and making it different to perform bodily functions that most of us take for granted. Those of you that know me well know that I don't like

talking about bodily functions, so let's leave this one right here.

So now the question becomes, what to do about it?

After I finished my final radiation treatment for the two initially identified spots, MD Anderson informed me, after a two-month wait, that I am not eligible for their PSMAfore clinical trial due to the presence of an AR V7 "splice variant" in my last Caris report. This is difficult to understand since that marker was readily identifiable in the Caris report previously received, but oh well. It is what it is.

This news means that I cannot rely on the Lu-177-PSMA-617 drug protocol to knock back the tumors in my rectal wall, so a different, more traditional strategy is needed. I met with my medical oncologist several times this week, and the current plan is that I will have a treatment port surgically inserted and will start chemotherapy with Taxotere.

Proving that God has a wicked sense of humor after all, it appears that I will lose some or most of my hair in the coming months. The hair is sometimes referred to by friends as the "pompadour" or the "man mane." Easy come, easy go. Oh well, at least I'm not whining... or am I?

BUBBLE BOY

AS I've mentioned before, if you spend any length of time around me, you will notice that I can barely get through a day without quoting (a) a line from some random movie; (2) a line from a song, or; (c) likening something that happened to something on an episode of Seinfeld. I still believe that every episode of "Seinfeld" was the best episode, so I had a good laugh yesterday when my medical oncologist told me that I am a "bubble boy," remembering something from one of my favorite Seinfeld episodes.

Perhaps I didn't really know what to expect with the first Taxotere infusion, but I was pleasantly surprised. Other than a little discomfort that came from "poking my port," there was almost nothing unpleasant about the experience. I want to pass along to anyone who might face this in the future that it did not hurt or burn, and it did not feel hot or cold. It was just "there." Start to finish, the process took about three hours. It was the first of six treatments that if things go as scheduled, will take place every three weeks until completion.

I do notice some side effects from the first treatment, none of which are profound. For instance, my tongue feels a little "weird," but it has not affected my sense of taste at this point (i.e. donuts and cinnamon rolls still taste good). I do feel tired — especially at night — but I run at a pretty hard pace, especially right now with so many things going on simultaneously at Cincinnati Cancer Advisors, so that might be contributing to the fatigue as well. I haven't lost any hair yet, though I am told that might not start until after treatment #2.

There is one significant side effect that is being addressed right now though. I had my first post- chemo blood work yesterday and my Absolute Neutrophil Count ("ANC") has dropped to near undetectable levels. ANC is basically a measure of the body's white blood cell count and is generally indicative of its ability to ward off infection, of which I have very little at the moment.

Therefore, I have to hunker down and do three very important things until the situation improves:

1. As soon as it is approved, return to the hospital for a Neulasta injection.
2. Do not leave my residential "bubble" for anything other than medical treatment and receive no guests.
3. Run — don't walk — to the ER if I begin to feel sick.

Now that I think of it, I am pretty sure none of this was ever addressed in an episode of Seinfeld.

YOU SOUND LIKE A REAL ATTRACTIVE GUY

SADLY, many people reading this might be too young to either remember Gilda Radner — one of the greatest comic talents in the '70s and '80s. Gilda died tragically in 1989 from ovarian cancer at the young age of 42. Despite that, she left us with some hilarious characters and comedic bits from "Saturday Night Live," including "Rosanne Rosannadanna."

This was one of my favorite Rosanne Rosannadanna bits from SNL's "Weekend Update":

A Mr. Richard Feder from Fort Lee, New Jersey, writes in and says "Dear Rosanne Rosannadanna, Last Thursday, I quit smoking. Now, I'm depressed, I get wet, my face broke out, I'm nauseous, I'm constipated, my feet swell, my gums are bleeding, my sinuses are clogged, I got heartburn, I'm cranky, and I have gas. What should I do?"

Mr. Feder you sound like a real attractive guy. You BELONG in New Jersey!

As it turns out, some of my favorite people are from New Jersey (you know who you are, Betty & Frank Carillo and Kevin Mooney). But I gotta tell ya... I feel a bit like a Mr. Richard Feder from New Jersey right about now because I never realized how much quitting smoking sounds like getting chemotherapy. With a few extra, added benefits thrown in for good measure.

For starters, I admit being vain about my hair and I am distressed about losing it, but maybe not for all of the reasons you might suspect. I am working wherever possible and prefer to do that in the company of other people, but it's embarrassing to sit next to someone while your hair appears to be falling out of your head at the same rate as our modern-day stock market. I'm self-conscious about it, which causes me to draw attention to it in an awkward way.

I noticed today that some of my fingernails are starting to turn an odd shade of purple. Without the benefit of nail polish, that is hard to hide. I have a big bump sticking out of my neck (my chemo port) like the bolt in Frankenstein's head that is pretty apparent whenever I wear a t-shirt or polo shirt. Oh, and I hiccup regularly for the two to three days after chemo. Apparently, all this is not that uncommon, and some people even require medication to put a stop to hiccups during chemotherapy. Who knew?

Last, I roam the halls at night. I went to bed at 7:45 p.m. tonight because I was exhausted after a long workday, and I am back up at 1:15 a.m. writing this and eating a bowl of Cinnamon Cheerios (I ate half of a baked potato and two forkfuls of corn before going to bed tonight). Please pray for my wife —she has been through this before as well and understands the side effects.

ROPE-A-DOPE

ONE definition of "Rope-A-Dope" is "a boxing tactic of pretending to be trapped against the ropes, goading an opponent to throw tiring, ineffective punches." Back before I questioned why grown adults were trying to knock one another out, I loved boxing. And I loved Muhammad Ali (I was just young enough to not ever know him as Cassius Clay).

I vaguely remember the lead-up to the "Rumble in the Jungle", the title match between Muhammad Ali and George Foreman (a fearsome heavyweight with devastating punching power before he transformed into a cheerful guy selling grills on QVC). Ali was never a massive physical presence, but he was a physical specimen. Truly one of the greatest boxers ever, he came up with the "rope-a-dope" as a strategy to let the other guy tire himself out, then overcome him with a combination of finesse and power. It was a brilliant strategy that helped propel Ali through one of the greatest and most successful periods in boxing history.

In a weird sort of way, when fighting cancer, the cancer patient also employs the rope-a-dope approach. For nearly a decade now, I have been doing things to try to understand what the opponent (i.e., cancer) is going to do next and in turn, what I need to do to offset it.

The first step was surgery. The thinking at the time was that surgery might... *might*... deal a devastating blow to a prostate cancer that already seemed to be more progressed than it should have been at my age. Surgery did not prevail, but I had a period where the impacts on my active lifestyle were minimal. All things being equal, and despite the ultimate outcome, I felt like I had won round one.

But then my PSA started to rise, potentially indicating an increase in disease volume. Four months after surgery, I began a series of 33 radiation treatments that were expected to knock prostate cancer to the mat. It didn't. I lost round two.

For the next six years, I began a series of "hormone" therapies that deprive a man's body of testosterone, one of the main fuels that prostate cancer uses to survive and thrive. There were ebbs and flows... relatively quick declines in PSA followed by relatively quick increases in PSA. For rounds 3-10, I had a plan, and it was working pretty well. Until it wasn't any more.

Now I am doing chemo, which appears to be working well. My PSA has dropped from 31 to 13, which is a good sign. Ironically enough, the accumulation of dead cancer cells can contribute to blood clots, which I experienced on a superficial basis this past weekend. It seems to always be something.

Cancer always seems to have an answer, but so do I and so do my doctors. The rope-a-dope is not a cure, but it's working. Survive and advance. Outlast and outperform. Envision your outcome and work towards it.

STEVE ABBOTT

NO REST FOR THE WICKED

OUR world is always busy as modern life dictates change and adaptation, while family and friends provide us meaning and support. Although my work and health care regimen was ongoing, I did escape to Belize with a group of my dearest people to celebrate my 60th birthday. Despite the title of this chapter, I had a very happy, restful time discovering a relatively new country in Central America. Belize celebrated their 41st year of independence in 2023 (they used to be called "British Honduras") and it still struggles as a decidedly third-world country. Those who greeted us there were some of the warmest people I have ever had the pleasure to know. We felt welcomed and appreciated and we all had a great time.

Returning home is always a whirlwind as well. The day after returning, I had a consultation with my radiation oncologist and received an injection of Eligard, a hormone therapy drug that clamps down on the production of testosterone in the testes (circulating testosterone generally feeds the growth of cancer cells so this is designed to starve the cancer cells of that fuel).

The following day brought the PSMA PET scan, a test I've had run three times before — twice in Michigan and once at MD Anderson. What's fantastic is that the PSMA PET scan can now be run in the Greater Cincinnati area, saving travel time and cost.

What is a PSMA PET scan, you ask?

The PSMA PET scan is still a relatively new tool in the cancer imaging toolkit. Oftentimes, prostate cancer cells have a "membrane" on their surface that is unique to prostate cancer cells. The PSMA PET scan relies on the "uptake" of a radioactive tracer by those prostate cancer cells, which causes them to light up, revealing their location. This type of precision in detecting prostate cancer was not readily available until recently, so it's kind of a big deal.

My PSMA PET scan results - meh. They could have been much better, but they also could have been much worse. The cancerous spots that were noted on my PSMA PET scan in April are still there, but most of those are smaller in size. There were a few new spots noted, but the hope is that maybe those are false positives that do not truly represent new areas of disease.

The bottom line: my level of improvement is substandard after four cycles of Taxotere, so on the advice of my medical oncologist, I scheduled an appointment at MD Anderson following my final chemo treatment in mid-October. The goal of that visit is to figure out the next treatment steps since the small improvement from the chemo is not expected to last very long, if at all. So as a line from one of my favorite Cage the Elephant songs goes, *ain't no rest for the wicked!*

STEVE ABBOTT

FANCY MEETING YOU HERE

WHEN I wrote the last chapter, the only thing I knew for certain is that che-motherapy won't be sufficient to control cancer in my case. Prostate cancer is still being found in my neck, chest, abdomen, and pelvis, with a few new areas of disease noted as well.

Aggressive disease does not benefit from a passive response so we needed to figure out what to do next.

In one of those "things that make you go *hmmm*" moments, I was able to meet my medical oncologist from MD Anderson (Dr. Christopher Logothetis) for dinner in Cincinnati. He is a highly sought-after speaker on genitourinary cancers who spoke at CCA's second annual "ASCO Direct Best of Oncology Highlights Conference".

Dinner provided a golden opportunity to discuss some details of my case and collect his initial thoughts on what to do next. It was very productive and in fact, my radiologic oncologist here in Cincinnati (i.e., Dr. Bill Barrett) is working on getting a copy of the disc from my most recent PSMA PET scan done in Cincinnati sent to MD Anderson so they can do a side-by-side compar-ison with the scan I had done in Texas in April.

Although the dinner meeting was planned, what happened that weekend wasn't. My local medical oncologist was also at the same conference, so these two were able to meet for the first time and discuss my case directly. Although there were many coincidences that led to this impromptu meeting, Drs. Bhan-dari and Logothetis are now collaborating on what might be coming next.

But wait, not so fast! I need some biopsies of the tissue in the affected areas, which will be a bit more invasive and add some time to my next stay in Hous-ton. This will give the docs a "molecular profile" that will tell them whether I am a potential candidate for Phase II clinical trials involving the use of a (*wait for it...*) PSMA-targeting bispecific antibody. This is a form of immunotherapy that has been shown to be effective at inducing antitumor responses against blood-based cancers. The hope is that this type of therapy will also prove to be effective against solid tumors like prostate cancer.

The last thing Dr. Logothetis did before he went back to Houston was that he put his hand on my shoulder and said to me, "Don't worry — we are going to take care of this." I don't know what the future holds but I do know two things: (1) I am going to learn a lot more about Houston, and (2) there is no substitute for hope when fighting cancer.

STEVE ABBOTT

A FUNNY THING HAPPENED ON
THE WAY TO THE BIOPSY

62

WOW, as much as I enjoy documenting this progress, I can't believe it's been five months since I last wrote the previous chapter of my cancer journey. So much has happened since then but, amazingly... almost unbelievably... not much has changed either.

When I last wrote, my four-month course of chemotherapy with Docetaxel had proven ineffective so my local medical oncologist was conferring with my medical oncologist at MD Anderson about how to proceed. There was evidence that the chemo had shrunk the tumors a bit, but not much, and it had not eliminated any of them. All the tumors were still where they were before, just a bit smaller.

From all of this, what had been decided was that I would go to MD Anderson for a tissue biopsy. The site of the biopsy would be my "supraclavicular node," an oversized lymph node near my neck in which prostate cancer cells were known to reside. Tissue "cores" would be taken and sent off to the lab for immediate processing to assess the stability of the tumor. This was chosen as the biopsy site because it was assumed to represent the overall molecular profile of my cancer, and because this bit of cancer was much easier to get to than the other sites (e.g., abdomen, lung, rectal wall).

But a funny thing happened on the way to the biopsy...

In the shower, I noticed that my left foot was enlarged. I asked Diana if it was just my imagination. No, she agreed that it was clearly enlarged and that I needed to get it checked. As (good) luck would have it, I already had a meeting scheduled with my radiation oncologist that afternoon. I asked him to look at it and without hesitation, he said "that is suspicious for a DVT," another way of saying a deep vein thrombosis, or a blood clot. Further analysis revealed that I had in fact developed three blood clots in my left leg but thankfully, they were not believed to be of the type that would break off and travel to my lungs.

Despite that, the trip to Houston was off since I was not able to fly or drive long distances in a car with unresolved blood clots. The visit to MD Anderson was not able to be rescheduled for an additional two months. That biopsy ultimately determined that my tumors were stable enough that there was minimal risk of starting a new therapy called Pluvicto, having things go south with my cancer, and then having to endure a "washout period" to get the Pluvicto out of my body before starting a new form of treatment.

Following my second bout with blood clots since starting chemotherapy, I am now on blood thinners and will be for the foreseeable future. Now I just need to get approved for Pluvicto. More on that later.

STEVE ABBOTT

AND SO IT BEGINS

SURVIVE *and* ADVANCE

SEPTEMBER — the start of prostate cancer awareness month, that is. It's been so long since I wrote the previous chapter so I just checked, and it was almost six months ago! And wow, has it been a busy six months!

But first things first... the start of prostate cancer awareness month. I am fortunate enough to have a few media appearances lined up to help get a message out that I really want to emphasize this year. The main points are:

1. There is no substitute for early detection of prostate cancer. Caught early, prostate cancer is almost always curable.
2. In my opinion, and my opinion only, if you are over 40 years of age with a family history that includes prostate cancer, there is no excuse for not at *least* getting a baseline PSA via a simple blood test.
3. Even if you don't catch prostate cancer early — and it's not curable — it is at least treatable. The advanced imaging techniques and targeted treatment options now available offer more hope and better outcomes than ever before.

Two weeks into September, I hope to make these points on Cincinnati's WLWT News. On a different TV station, our best known local health reporter and I are planning another segment in September to cover the success I am currently enjoying with Pluvicto, a targeted radioligand treatment that I started five months earlier.

So yes, Pluvicto. When I last wrote, I had been approved to start treatment with Pluvicto but it was not available. Like not available anywhere in the U.S. Novartis had started production but had to halt when they self-reported quality control problems to the Food & Drug Administration.

Guys that had started on the treatment — which was the next big hope for those with advanced prostate cancer — suddenly had problems accessing it. Many, if not most, who had been approved for the treatment (including me) were informed that they were on hold, and there was no indication as to when the situation would be resolved. Meanwhile, PSAs were increasing, along with the stress level of tens of thousands of men around the country that needed to start on the treatment to control their cancer. It was a mess.

After waiting several months, I "got the call" and was told that I would receive my first Pluvicto treatment the next week. A week later, I got another call... this one was from my treatment provider, telling me that my treatments were being canceled... ALL of them... because the reimbursement from my insurance coverage was going to fall a few hundred dollars short for each treatment. Stay tuned.

65

STEVE ABBOTT

YOU'VE GOT TO BE KIDDING ME

ONLY a week before I was scheduled to start treatment with Pluvicto, I received a phone call from a representative of my treatment provider saying, "I have some bad news." Right away, I knew that she was going to tell me that the treatment was still not available, and I'd have to wait longer to start treatment. I said that to her and she said, "I actually wish that is why I was calling you."

I laughed and said something like what could be worse than that? She very nervously informed me that she had to cancel my treatments altogether. After waiting for months, I was more than a little frustrated and asked her why they were canceling me if it wasn't due to supply problems with the treatment. She told me that they had received word from my insurance company that the reimbursement for each treatment was going to be $850 less than what they needed to move forward with it. This, on a treatment that costs $45,000 per dose.

I said, "you've GOT to be kidding me." She said, "I wish I was." I asked whether this was just a timing thing... like maybe it was being delayed while they worked out the reimbursement details with the insurance company. She told me that it wasn't — that they couldn't make money at the level of reimbursement they were going to be receiving. That's it. End of story. Cancelled. Go somewhere else? Not as easy as it sounds. This provider was the only place nearby that had the treatment.

As it turns out, our local health reporter from Local 12 — Liz Bonis - had just filmed a story with me and my provider. The gist of the story was about the hope and promise that this new treatment offered to guys with advanced prostate cancer — guys whose treatment options were limited, short of a clinical trial. The story was just about "in the can" and ready to run on TV, so I immediately contacted Liz for two reasons: (1) so she could pull the story since I was apparently no longer going to be treated there and (2) in hopes she might be able to bring some pressure to bear.

She knocked the ball out of the park, asking them to either provide (a) a written statement as to why my treatments were being canceled or (b) have a member of their executive team go on camera explaining their decision. Within hours, I was contacted by the provider's CEO, telling me there had been a "mistake," and that my treatments were back on. Liz asked for a promise from them that they would follow through with all treatments and they said they would. Thankfully, they have stayed true to their word and I ended up receiving all six treatments.

By now, you might be wondering "what happens to people that don't have a TV reporter as their advocate in cases like this?" It's a valid question, and a troubling one. Stay tuned.

HURRY UP, AND WAIT

SO, now we are up to treatment day with Pluvicto... finally. But wait! Around 9:30 that morning, I got a phone call from my treatment provider. I saw it come up on the Caller ID and braced myself. Are they calling to cancel me again? Thankfully, no. Or at least not on purpose.

While Novartis' supply issues were beginning to improve, their production facility in New Jersey had still not been re-certified by the FDA. As such, Pluvicto treatments being administered in the U.S. were almost exclusively being produced at Novartis' manufacturing facility in Italy and shipped to the U.S. on a "just-in-time" basis for the treatment.

Anyway, my treatment provider was calling to tell me that my treatment was likely off for the day as the raw materials for the treatment had arrived in New Jersey, but still had to clear U.S. Customs and the FDA. My treatment was scheduled for 1:00 p.m. and under a best-case scenario, it was at least 2 ½ hours away by plane, even *if* it was approved immediately thereafter. Knowing that it still had to get from Cincinnati's international airport (located in Northern Kentucky) to their office, I figured it was hopeless and started making other plans for the day. The caller pretty much confirmed that was going to be the case, but she was holding out hope.

At about 12:15 p.m., I received a call from the same person saying that the treatment was "back on" and asking if I could still make it. Given that I was a solid 30 minutes away by car, I said "is it still a 1 o'clock appointment?" She confirmed that it was, and just asked me to do my best to get there as close to the start time as possible.

I made it there by 1:15 p.m. and was quickly ushered into the treatment room, which bordered on surreal. Given the radioactive payload that was about to be injected into my body, I was asked if I needed to go to the bathroom (they don't want you using the "facilities" following treatment). The bathroom was hilarious. Everything, and I mean everything, was wrapped in a thick layer of plastic. Handles, faucets, the toilet seat, the door handle, etc.

Now back in the room, I wondered aloud at how the treatment was in New Jersey as of 9:30 a.m. that day, and somehow cleared U.S. Customs and the FDA and still made it in time for a 1:00 p.m. treatment. Now, here comes the best part. As it turns out, it had been in their building all along — they just didn't know it. What a "cluster," as they say.

Once the treatment began, it was amazing at how quickly it went — completed in less than 10 minutes. After it was over, they "wanded" me with some sort of device which confirmed that I was "hot." I was told to go straight home and quarantine for several days.

HOT, HOT, HOT

SURVIVE *and* ADVANCE

AS I mentioned in the last chapter, the Pluvicto treatment was over in virtually no time. It's a fascinating if not daunting process though. There's always a team of at least three people in the room during the treatment; a radiation oncologist, a registered nurse, and a chemist. There is lots of communication back and forth between these three individuals throughout the treatment. All three must agree on each step before that step can take place. At the end of the treatment, the syringe is inspected to make sure that 99%+ of the toxic nectar made it into the patient.

I found it to be ironic, bordering on comical. It was such a struggle to get approved for the treatment and to access it, and in a matter of a few minutes, it was over. I can't say I felt anything at all during the injection. It didn't burn, and I didn't feel hot or cold, or anything unusual for that matter. I continue to marvel at the fact that liquid that fits in a medium-sized syringe could cost $45,000 per treatment, but I also recognize that the price has nothing to do with the liquid, but rather the years and years of research that went into developing the treatment. I give thanks every day for the scientists, medical professionals, and clinical trial participants that make treatment advances possible.

Once I was home, I began my three days of quarantine. Prior to starting treatment, I was called in for a briefing on the need to maintain distance from people — especially babies and pregnant women — for a period of about three days following treatment. Patients are strongly encouraged to use a separate bathroom since you will be "hot" and as such, need to maintain at least six feet of distance from other people to protect them from the radiation.

I am currently a decade deep into near-continuous treatment for advanced prostate cancer. My 60+-year-old body has been mutilated, castrated (chemically; not the other way thankfully!), medicated, irradiated, and deprived of essential hormones that regulate health and quality of life. Through surgery, multiple courses of radiation, seven years of hormone-altering drugs, chemotherapy and radiotherapy that requires that you not even been around people for days at a time, I feel fine. I do feel tired at times since I am now an out-of-shape 60 year old who doesn't eat or sleep well. But other than that, I rarely either notice - or choose to pay attention to - anything other than feeling fine. It amazes me, what the body can tolerate and either heal from, or compensate for.

But as for the side effects stemming from this new treatment, I woke the day following treatment feeling slightly nauseous and with a low-grade headache. As they say in the movies, these things were foretold to me. I took one Zofran and two Tylenol and within hours, I felt back to normal. This is going to be fine, I thought.

I WISH I COULD DROP MY GOLF SCORE LIFE THIS

SO, my treatment regimen with Pluvicto had finally been approved, secured, and begun. That was nearly five months ago and I have held off posting much in hopes that I would have good news to report. And boy, do I!

There is one bit of information that I need to share for context before I get into the good news. Historically, I have been a bit of an underperformer when it comes to treatment for advanced prostate cancer. If a certain type of treatment was supposed to buy a typical advanced prostate cancer guy five more years, I'd be lucky to get two out of it before my PSA would begin rising again. Oral treatments like Xtandi could typically be expected to be effective for two or more years, and I was failing at four months. Chemotherapy — pretty much the mother of all cancer treatments — was largely ineffective against my cancer.

Despite the treatment frustration that had built up over the years, I went into this Pluvicto treatment regimen with high hopes. My past experiences caused me to temper my enthusiasm ever so slightly, but I was also mindful of the many positive reports I had heard from medical oncologists about the effectiveness that Pluvicto was showing in early data.

To review just a bit, Pluvicto is what is referred to as a "radioligand" treatment. In practical terms, what it does is use a radiotracer (such as Gallium 68 or Pylarify) dispensed from either a tungsten or lead-based container,to locate the prostate cancer cells, and a radioisotope (in this case, Lutetium-177) to destroy those cancer cells. This is what they call a "PSMA- targeted treatment," as it can work in men that have a base layer protein called "PSMA" (prostate- specific membrane antigen) present on their prostate cancer cells. Thankfully, about 80% of men with prostate cancer do express this PSMA protein on their prostate cancer cells and can therefore benefit from the treatment.

So far, the data on treatment with Pluvicto has been great, showing not only a quantifiable life-extension benefit, but also good durability. That said, even amongst the guys that are "PSMA positive," only about 65%-70% will show an effective response. But it's a great start, and there will surely be additional PSMA-targeted treatments that will be coming along. Despite these limitations, Pluvicto appears to be — at the very least — a "game changer" in terms of prostate cancer control.

When I started treatment on April 21, 2023, my PSA was 25 and climbing. Since then — and remember, PSA is like golf... the lower the number, the better:

May 13, 2023	111.3
June 19, 2023	99.6
August 4, 2023	55.1
August 31, 2023	33.6
September 20, 2023	22.9

For a guy that has not had the best luck with treatment, these are STUNNING results and a good indication the treatment is working in my case. In my next post, I'll address what happens when my PSA (inevitably) starts to rise again.

❦

UNTOUCHABLE

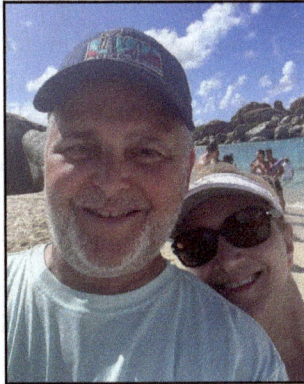

Steve & Diana at British Virgin Islands.

I have always loved to travel. So much so that it has been an obsession for me during most of my life. Diana has been a great companion throughout, although there were probably times when she might have preferred to stay home.

My zest for travel was forged early. We were a family of six. Like so many other families, my mother ran an amazingly efficient (and happy) household. My father worked as many jobs as it took to make sure that if we didn't always have what we wanted, we had at least what we needed.

One luxury that was non-negotiable back when I was growing up: our family always took a two-week vacation. Granted, this was the early 1970's. Airplane trips were only for "rich" people so our family vacations were always somewhere drivable from Northern Kentucky, generally to either Florida or South Carolina. The 14- to 24-hour drive tested the family's mettle, but I still look upon those trips as some of my favorite adventures.

We always were so excited about vacation. These trips didn't come easily to a family like ours, but we somehow managed to do it every year. To maximize our vacation time, we would leave after my father had worked a full day and we would then depart in the middle of the night, like the Von Trapp family escaping the Nazis in "The Sound of Music." If my father didn't think he could make it all the way to Florida, we'd stop somewhere along the way. There was no Google nor travel "apps" at the time. Think of it - six humans crammed into a single Holiday Inn room, but we made it work. We often had to stop at multiple motels to find one with a vacancy.

Back then, there were no cell phones and no "work from home." There was no expectation that you would "check in" with work during your travels. When you left on vacation, you were GONE AWAY - essentially unreachable and untouchable until you returned home.

By the time we left for vacation, my PSA was on the rise again. The second test confirmed that the first result was not a fluke. It was a huge disappointment because things had been going so well with my new treatment. But I was not surprised.

Today, while trying to keep the sea water out of my snorkel mask and snorkel tube — all the while observing hundreds of parrotfish, blue tang, and the occasional jellyfish — I felt untouchable by cancer. The need to discuss "next steps" with my oncology team will bring me back to reality soon enough but not today. For now, cancer is back home... almost 2,000 miles away... and not to be contemplated any further on this AMAZING trip.

IF AT FIRST YOU DON'T SUCCEED

UNFORTUNATELY, my PSA is on the rise again after nearly six months of precipitous decline while on Pluvicto. I've mentioned before the nervous anticipation experienced by cancer patients when waiting for test results. I would venture a guess that this anxiety affects all cancer patients because no matter how long ago you were diagnosed, or you've been told that "there is no evidence of disease," or "it looks like you are in remission," one never knows for sure. The rare exception is the one thing that all cancer patients dream of hearing: "you are considered cured."

Diana and I had such an amazing trip to the U.S. Virgin Islands. It was a "do-over" trip for us as we were both sick with respiratory infections when we went away six months prior. This trip could not have been more different. We both felt well and had one of the most active vacations we have had in a long time, taking several day-long snorkeling trips.

For the first time in 20+ years, we took a jet ski out for the afternoon. The jet ski was the most exhilarating and terrifying thing I have done in a long time. Diana is our daredevil whenever it comes to driving something. I have been more than happy to let her drive us, even around Rome in past trips to Italy, as she seems to prefer the stress of driving over the stress of having someone else control her destiny. So naturally, she took control of the jet ski and I held on for dear life.

Having only done this one time before, I had no idea that holding onto the handles on the back of the jet ski was a terrible choice relative to the better option, which was to wrap my arms around Diana's waist and hope for the best. For the first 20 minutes, the possibility of dying from cancer was the farthest thing from my mind since I thought there was a more likely chance that I would meet my demise on the back of that jet ski.

But now, back home, it's also back to real life, specifically, figuring out what to do about my rising PSA.

Speaking with my medical oncologist at MD Anderson, we have a new plan. I will go back to Houston for a PSMA PET scan and consult with him about "next steps." One possible option is to do targeted radiation on the tumors that remain post-Pluvicto.

Another option would be some sort of clinical trial like bispecific antibody treatment that could hopefully be done on an outpatient basis and allow me to commute to Houston rather than move there.

Dr. Logothetis' most recent text message to me said, "No worries. There is still plenty we can do," so I am going to roll with that.

THE MORE THINGS CHANGE,
THE MORE THEY STAY THE SAME

IT'S now Christmas Eve. After returning from MD Anderson, my post-Pluvicto PSA dropped to 2.95. There was a lot of high-fiving and back-slapping going on. I was the ringleader of those celebrations, feeling as if I'd finally found a treatment that would offer a durable, favorable response. In fact, there was every indication that would be the case.

But as they say... the more things change, the more they stay the same. October brought new information. Combined with my history, I knew right away that a rise in my PSA was a troubling development. My PSA was 3.30 a month later. Although my medical oncologist was not overly concerned, I already smelled a rat because I know what happens when my PSA starts to rise. It never rises slowly.

I know a PSA rise from 2.95 to 3.30 doesn't seem like much. For some folks, a PSA of 3.30 is not even a scary number. Oncologists are often more concerned about "PSA velocity" — that is, how quickly that number rises - than they are about the raw PSA number. On November 8, 2023, my PSA was 3.68; on December 4, 2023, it was 5.80, and it jumped to 7.30 on December 9, 2023. These are alarming increases in PSA over a very short time, especially following what had been precipitous declines in PSA while on Pluvicto.

I had an updated PSMA PET scan in Houston. The "PSMA PET" is a game-changing diagnostic imaging tool that was not FDA-approved or widely available as recently as the beginning of 2022. Prior to the PSMA PET scan, it was very difficult, if not impossible, for oncologists to identify with certainty where prostate cancer cells reside. Without that information, targeted treatments were not really a "thing." This new imaging technique now provides precise information to oncology teams that allow for more effective and in some cases, less invasive treatments.

The good news is that Pluvicto did its job. The scan told us that all previously existing disease sites are now smaller in size. However, it also identified bone metastasis for the first time in my spine at vertebrae L2 and T8. Coincidentally, my back has been way screwed up for months, so much so that I could barely get out of bed. Although the PSMA PET scan can't tell me whether the back problems I am experiencing are related to cancer, it now seemed hard to rule it out given the timing.

So now I wait for an updated treatment plan from the team at MD Anderson. I don't know the details yet, but I was told while there that there's no time to wait... that whatever we end up doing, we need to start ASAP. So once again, I'll blow through my annual deductible and maximum out-of-pocket medical expense in January. Here we go!

THIS IS WHY I WRITE

ONE of my favorite songs from the last decade (or two) is called *"This is Why We Fight"* by The Decemberists. In the early days of my cancer diagnosis, I thought I would adopt it as my fight song... something I could listen to loudly in the car on the way to work in order to get mentally ready to take on another day.

I was addicted to the melody, vocals, and instrumentation of the song but I couldn't figure out its words or meaning. I looked up the lyrics and it looked like a bunch of gibberish to me but nonetheless, I thought (and still think) it's a very cool song. Meanwhile, it occurred to me recently that it might be worth re-explaining why I write this blog in the first place. So, without further ado (and with deference to The Decemberists), *this is why I write:*

1. Because I have always enjoyed it, and still do. From writing for my high school newspaper to creative writing classes in high school and college, it just always felt comfortable for me. However, a career consisting mostly of accounting and finance roles didn't leave much room for that.

2. I was diagnosed with cancer in August 2013 and by January 2014, I knew it was an advanced form of the disease. I decided at that time to do whatever I could to help other cancer patients and writing about my experience was one way to do that.

3. Although my goal is to do my best to help all cancer patients, I have a particular interest in talking to people about prostate cancer — because it is **so curable** when caught early. Said another way, for most guys, there is no reason to die of prostate cancer (although sadly, 35,000 American men still do each year).

4. People for whom I have immense respect — like my friend Donna Salyers (who was recently named a "Great Living Cincinnatian") have told me that I should "write a book someday." Strangely enough, this blog turned into this short book...written 500 words at a time.

As a reminder, my blog is named *"5 Years; 500 Words at a Time."* I gave it that name for two reasons:

1. My goal was to live at least five more years with advanced prostate cancer. If so, that would mean I lived 13-14 years with advanced cancer. I still wouldn't be ready to leave at that point, but that would be a pretty good accomplishment.

2. 500 words gives you enough space to say some things, make a point or two, ramble a bit at times (but not too much), and close each entry out before you bore the **** out of people.

How amazing would it be if you could string a bunch of blog entries together into a book and perhaps help people by showing that in some cases, living well with cancer is possible? Maybe I'll do that someday.

40 IS THE NEW 50

AS previously mentioned, two tests — a spinal MRI in combination with the PSMA PET scan — conclusively determined that the cancer had progressed to my bones. In this case, cancer was found in vertebrae L2 and T8, which explained the intense back pain I had been experiencing during the last four months. The scan revealed "pathologic compression fractures" in my spine.

With reckless disregard for the advice I gave in *"The Median is Not the Message,"* of course, I immediately looked up pathologic compression fractures and found that they are "associated with end stage cancer" with "high morbidity and mortality". According to the website I found, 30%-40% of people with pathologic compression fractures make it one year following diagnosis.

For the first time in a long time, I let some random website ruin my day. It was a mental setback that took consultations with my wife, my mother, my doctor, and a few glasses of wine to overcome. But I did indeed overcome it, and now re-emphasize that your life is your life... it's not a bundle of statistics that predict your demise off some random website.

Nonetheless, I am using it as jet fuel to feel better because on June 9, 2024, Diana and I will celebrate our 40th wedding anniversary. Given the current landscape with respect to outcomes for advanced prostate cancer patients who have failed nearly every available, FDA-approved therapy, I do not expect to be here for my 50th wedding anniversary. I hope I am (pardon the pun) dead wrong about that but in the meantime, I am going to use it as an excuse to plan an amazing trip for our 40th wedding anniversary.

When booking our first-ever trip to France, we splurged for the flat bed "Delta One" seats (tonic for my aching back). Four nights in Paris, followed by four nights on the French Riviera (well, Monaco if you want to split hairs). As a lifelong tennis fan, I'd love to get to Roland Garros for a day at the French Open — maybe I will, or maybe not. But it's all good. (note: Diana spent the day after our wedding as a tennis widow as I watched the French Open in our honeymoon suite in Charleston, SC some forty years prior).

I'm not a gambler but I won't miss the opportunity to hang out in the casino in Monte Carlo, site of cool James Bond movies I used to watch with my parents. We will do it up in France because... as they say... 40 is the new 50!

WHISTLING PAST
THE GRAVEYARD

SURVIVE and ADVANCE

I'VE always loved and been amused by this phrase, that is, "to act or talk as if one is relaxed and not afraid... when one is actually afraid or nervous; to show a confident manner, but actually may just be *whistling past the graveyard*."

One of the kindest compliments I receive from people these days regards my "positivity," "optimism," and "attitude." It's not an act, but it is a conscious choice at times. There are lots of ups and downs that come with cancer, especially with advanced cancer (where cancer has spread to a distant part of the body, or beyond the primary cancer site).

Thankfully, it's been a fairly long journey for me so far, over a decade of no notable period of remission and no real break from continuous treatment. Lots of test results along the way. I jokingly celebrate with Diana any week that doesn't involve poking, prodding, or a "needlestick" of some sort. Each result involves a high five, a shoulder shrug, or an "oh, ****."

One of the things that has allowed me to primarily maintain a positive attitude throughout is that I have rarely "felt sick" to this point. Even the rigors of chemotherapy were not as bad as I thought they were going to be. Radiation (eight times in ten years, no less!) has been a comparative breeze. Eight years of hormone therapy has left me with a soft, huggable, lumpy body and a respectable "B cup" (those that wear a bra will understand).

Despite the treatment-related side effects, I have rarely *felt* as if I have cancer in my body. I have always known it was there... the numbers and the scans tell me that and often show it. But I have rarely *felt* it until recently. The constant, cancer-related, lower back pain I have experienced lately has presented a bit more of a challenge. But a few courses of steroids have helped get the inflammation down and have made me feel more like my old self. It makes a huge difference in your attitude when you don't "feel" it as much. It also gives me a great appreciation for other cancer patients and people with debilitating diseases that are not so fortunate.

People often confuse "palliative care" with hospice or end-of-life care, whereas it really refers to specialized care that helps mitigate pain and other symptoms resulting from serious, often incurable, disease. For the first time in my life, I am seriously considering "talking to somebody" (a Steve euphemism for talking to a "therapist"). I have done a good job of staying one step ahead of this disease from a physical standpoint, but I anticipate some treatment anxiety when it comes to starting immunotherapy, which is still a bit choppy and unpredictable when it comes to prostate cancer. I just need to find the time to do that, because the mental part of managing this disease is also important.

I'LL SLEEP WHEN I'M DEAD

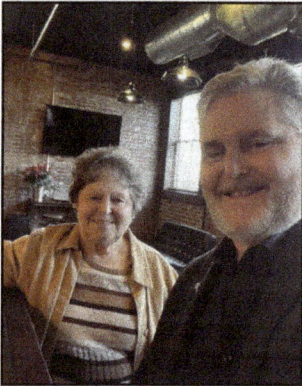

Steve and his mother, Barbara Abbott, enjoying a bourbon tasting at Peerless Distilling in Louisville, Kentucky.

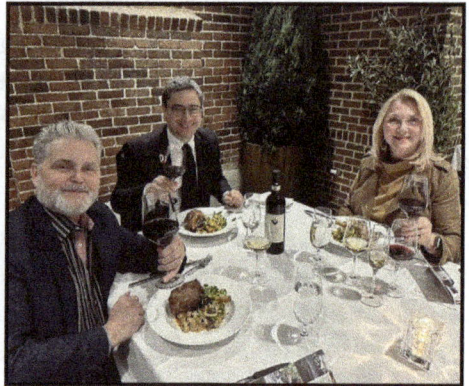

Steve and Diana with the winemaker and owner of Bocale Winery, Valentino Valentini, at Lytle Park Hotel in Cincinnati, Ohio.

SURVIVE *and* ADVANCE

ONE of my favorite Warren Zevon songs is *"I'll Sleep When I'm Dead."* It was also a saying of my very colorful, dearly departed maternal grandmother, Joy Smith. It's also a mantra of mine.

It's been an absolute whirlwind since my last chapter six weeks ago, as this morning's review of my calendar will attest. I knew the pace didn't really leave me time to write, but the following list gives a bit more insight into why:

- Interview with Local 12's Liz Bonis and my colleague Sherry Hughes for a show called *"Cancer Breakthroughs."*
- Met with an NFL Hall of Famer ?? to discuss fundraising initiatives for Cincinnati Cancer Advisors.
- Began and completed radiation to eradicate the cancer found in my L2 vertebrae.
- Interviews on FOX 19 and KISS 107.1's *"Jon, Jon & Friends"* to discuss the importance of World Cancer Day.
- Took my mother on a weekend bourbon tasting adventure to the mecca, aka Louisville, Kentucky.
- Filmed three Cincinnati Cancer Advisors *"Medical Minute"* podcasts.
- Participated with my colleagues over three days to host the first of two *"Wine, Women & Shoes"* fundraising events this year for our cancer charity.
- Completed a separate course of radiation to eradicate the cancer found in my T8 vertebrae.
- Four days of filming and speaking at a pharmaceutical conference in Orlando, Florida where Diana and I had an opportunity to tell our story as cancer survivors, and advocate on behalf of other cancer survivors.
- Attended a spectacular wine dinner with the owner of Bocale Winery from Umbria, Italy.
- Attended the Greater Cincinnati Chamber of Commerce dinner where our great Cincinnati Cancer Advisors supporter John Barrett and my dear friend Donna Salyers were honored as "Great Living Cincinnatians."
- Spoke at an *"Innovation in Oncology"* dinner where I was honored to meet John and Liza Marshall, authors of *"Off Our Chests,"* and speak on the shared experience that Diana and I have as both cancer survivors and caregivers.

This above is just a partial list from the past six weeks. Not on the list is the ZERO Prostate Cancer Summit in Washington, D.C., where nearly 150 prostate cancer advocates "storm the hill" to request increased funding for prostate cancer research. I normally participate every year, but I was not feeling well enough to tromp around Capitol Hill this year. Next year for sure, though.

I need to slow things down, but I feel very fortunate to be busy, and still relevant, at the ripe old age of 61. At an age when people often begin to feel "invisible," I am privileged to have the opportunity to speak regularly about things I am passionate about. I meet amazing people every single week.

In the filming session we had a few weeks ago, we talked about how TERRIFIED I used to be when it came to any form of public speaking. Cancer changed that for me. I was not symptomatic, yet I had advanced cancer at diagnosis. I feel an obligation to warn others about that possibility.

IT'S BETTER TO LOOK GOOD
THAN TO FEEL GOOD

THERE are many TV shows that I've always been a sucker for. Diana right-fully calls me a "news junkie" since the morning news is the first thing I turn on upon waking. No day is complete unless I have watched at least 2-3 hours of news programming in the evening.

I have always been addicted to other programs as well and have recently added a new addiction: *Curb Your Enthusiasm* (just in time for it to end its 12-season run).

Other notable "favorite" addictions over the years have been college basketball, *Entourage, Seinfeld* and of course, *Saturday Night Live*, which I watched faithfully ever since my parents first let me start watching it. There have been amazing casts, unbelievably talented performers...as well as quite a few forgettable seasons along the way. One of those largely forgettable seasons was the 1+ year that comedian Billy Crystal was a working member of the SNL cast.

Despite a largely forgettable and short run, Billy had one recurring sketch that still makes me laugh to this day, which was his parody of Fernando La-mas and his "it's better to look good than to feel good" line. As absurd as that sounds, there is something to be said for getting up every day and putting your-self together as best you can, even on the days when you don't feel good. I recall my grandmother Joy Smith, who battled heart disease and diabetes for many years before her eventual passing, applying her many layers of makeup each morning and wearing a wig so she always looked as good as she could. She was a very proud woman.

Lately, it feels like my cancer is starting to break through the sandbags I have thrown down to stop its progress over the last decade. Until very recently, ongoing treatment was a necessary nuisance, but my body felt surprisingly re-silient throughout. Surgery, radiation (more times than I can count), hormone deprivation therapy for more than eight years, and even chemotherapy felt like comparatively small physical setbacks in the grand scheme of things.

Success to date has been defined by keeping the cancer out of my bones and organs. The frustrating pace with which cancer is now invading my spine, accompanied by the pain, is now being complicated by the first signs of kidney problems. It's a concerning new chapter with broad implications for my ability to fight this disease.

Quite frankly, I am worried about it. But life goes on. Spring now hangs in the balance and "March Madness" has begun. Soon my TV will be filled with images of screaming fans and the strains of exuberant commentators celebrating "buzzer beaters" as David upsets Goliath during the most exciting tournament in sports. For Goliath, all that's needed is to survive, and advance, whereas the upstart teams needs only to put together one game where they play above the rim and knock off the favorite.

For now, my goal is to keep up appearances, keep putting one foot in front of the other, and hang tough until I both look better AND feel better. It's certainly what Joy Smith would have done.

STEVE ABBOTT

MARCH MADNESS —
THE STRUGGLE IS REAL!

A bit of unvarnished honesty to start. The two weeks since I last wrote have largely sucked, but I'm still standing (or at least trying to sit comfortably).

First, March Madness. It's well underway and my beloved Kentucky Wildcats — once again — have managed to exit both the SEC and NCAA tournaments in embarrassing fashion by losing in the first round of both tournaments (note: this would represent the beginning-of-the-end for Hall of Fame UK coach John Calipari). My bracket is now more busted than my back feels. There are no local teams left, but there are still a few "Cinderellas" at the dance to root for (go North Carolina State!).

Meanwhile, the only way I could have spent more time running back and forth to the hospital in the last two weeks is if I worked there. When I last wrote, I made mention of seeing the early signs of kidney problems. My spinal MRI had revealed something called "hydronephrosis" on my right side. Hydronephrosis is when something prevents urine (I hate talking about this stuff) from flowing properly between the kidneys and the bladder, from where it exits the body.

The suspicion was that a kidney stone was the culprit, especially since small kidney stones have shown up for several years on my scans. I wasn't having pain though. As people who have had kidney stones before (myself included) will attest, there is usually associated pain.

Because of what we saw on my scan, and what was suspected, I was referred for bloodwork, which showed a higher-than-normal creatinine level and a lower-than-normal eGFR (the eGFR is typically a pretty reliable indicator of kidney function). Despite 10+ years of fighting cancer, this had never happened before.

I made an appointment with a urologist, who almost immediately ruled out kidney stone as a cause. He was notably concerned and scheduled a renal scan to "get under the hood" and figure out what was going on. In the meantime, he referred me for additional bloodwork, which revealed a further, rapid, and precipitous decline in my kidney function. My eGFR had dropped to 28 (a normal range for a 60-year-old man would be closer to 60-90) and at the rate my kidneys were failing, there was legitimate concern about having to go on kidney dialysis in short order. The renal scan was canceled, and emergency surgery to install two renal stents was scheduled.

Now... if you have no idea what any of this means... and if you have never heard of the term "ureter" or "stent" and don't know what ureters do — good for you, please keep it that way! As it turns out, the blockages in my ureters were caused by scar tissue that was the result of past radiation to my pelvis and abdomen over the past decade. At the time, it was necessary to keep the cancer at bay, so what are you going to do?

With cancer, you fight the biggest fight in front of you and worry about the rest later. But for the first time, it feels like cancer might be winning.

WELCOME TO MY NIGHTMARE

I had the sounds of Alice Cooper's *"Welcome to My Nightmare"* bouncing around in my head when I wrote the last entry. You see, now cancer is messing around with the most private and sensitive part(s) of my body (Google "how is a renal stent inserted on a man" and you'll see what I am referring to. Not fun.).

Diana will tell you how modest I am about things like this. I think back to high school gym class. One hour of running, or playing dodge ball or basketball, followed by the dreaded group shower. I never knew which to be more horrified of... contracting "athlete's foot" from the shower floor or being in a group shower with ten other dudes. Ugh.

The thought of having two thin plastic tubes shoved "up there" did not sit very well with me going into the surgery. In fact, I was horrified. But failing kidneys and being strapped to a dialysis machine sounded way worse, so into the operating room we go!

Prostate cancer yields many surprises for the guys that have it. You have probably read of the various side effects that come with treatment, none of which are anything you would choose. What you don't often read about is what ten years of treatment — prostate gland removal, radiation, and hormone (i.e. testosterone) deprivation — do to the male "anatomy." I can tell you that it's not good! So, if I wasn't self-conscious before, I sure am now.

But hey, it is what it is. I reported to the hospital for the procedure three hours early for (a) my daily radiation treatment for the cancer in my L3 vertebrae and (b) "pre-op." Good times indeed. Plenty of time to lay there and dread what was coming next. Thankfully, my high school sweetheart and wife of forty years was by my side the whole time.

While waiting for surgery, we talked about how miraculous it is that we live in a time where blood work can identify a major problem, imaging techniques can identify the *exact* location of that problem, anesthesia can keep you from feeling pain or remembering the procedure used to rectify that problem, and there are skilled, trained professionals that can use little robotic arms to insert or remove things from your body with minimal collateral damage. It's truly fascinating.

Finally, the time for my surgery drew near. My surgeon came in to talk to me about the procedure, telling me he was hopeful and optimistic that the stents could be placed and that they would work. The alternative was that I would wake up with a nephrostomy tube. I had enough time to Google "nephrostomy tube" before surgery. Are you kidding me? How did we *get* here? A nephrostomy sounds absolutely terrible.

So now it's go-time. I jokingly told my surgeon that he might need a Hubble telescope to do his work today. He is of Indian descent. I am American. Thankfully, despite any cultural differences between us, the joke landed. We all laughed, and that's the last thing I remember about the surgery.

ONE THING AFTER ANOTHER, PART II

AFTER the last few weeks, I feel like I've earned the right to be lazy and re-use one of my previous chapter titles, especially since it applies in this case. In the last chapter, I relayed an anecdote of a joke I made when I was going into my surgery. English is not the first language of my surgeon, so it could have bombed, but it transcended our two languages and was a welcome way to cut the tension.

We've all heard over the years about the differences between British and American humor. Colloquialisms often don't work across languages, or the accents can make it difficult to even understand in the first place (cockney comes to mind). British humor, in my judgment, tends to be more slapstick in nature than American humor, evoking an almost vaudeville approach to comedy that I don't always love. But a good sight gag always works and transcends languages. One such example is from one of my favorite movies of all time — *"Monty Python & the Holy Grail."*

There is a hilarious scene where two hapless soldiers are guarding a castle gate. They see Sir Lancelot running toward them, for what seems like an eternity, but he never seems to get any closer. This goes on for a bit, then suddenly, he's upon them and they are overrun by this single foe. It is a hilarious sight gag that feels very much like how my cancer journey has gone recently.

As mentioned in a previous chapter *("Rope-A-Dope"),* this whole battle has been a series of punches and counter punches, with cancer throwing the punches while my oncology team figures out how to respond. All therapeutic responses, though rarely optimal, have been effective in kicking the can down the road and buying more time. It's easy to underestimate the importance of that, but it has literally added time to my life where new discoveries have come along, and I have been able to avail myself of those treatments.

I previously shared that it felt like cancer was starting to win. This was obviously disappointing, but it was a real emotion at the time. The recent placement of the renal stents were urgent in nature, done in response to a potentially life-threatening situation, and were the direct result of previous counter punches to the cancer — i.e., necessary radiation to my abdomen and pelvis.

I am happy to report that I seem to be adjusting to the renal stents relatively well. The bladder spasms — which occurred often in the aftermath of the surgery — were both regular and painful. Those are occurring less often now; it hurts much less to urinate than in the days immediately following the procedure.

I had to stop taking the blood thinners for the procedure. I am on blood thinners permanently now due to having an active cancer case, which can contribute to the development of blood clots. (I have read articles suggesting that cancer patients — on average — are nine times more likely to develop blood clots than those without cancer). I was only off the blood thinners for four days for this procedure (which was necessary to control the risk of excess bleeding) and — lo and behold — I developed a blood clot in my left leg, my third such blood clot. Hopefully, that has now fully resolved.

A mental adjustment is now seeing blood in my urine, regularly, and in fairly significant amounts. My red blood counts are low as a result, but not low enough to require blood transfusions to this point. Hopefully it stays that way, and hopefully the bleeding stops soon. It's hard not to worry about it, as it's not at all normal.

Like I said, it's been one damn thing after another.

NEXT STEPS

SO... what next? I have completed radiation on the cancer found in three separate vertebrae — L2, L3 and T8. Radiation to L1 will commence at some point, but not now. The radiation was intended to relieve some, if not all of the back pain. Has it? Not really.

My new regimen is trying to calibrate the minimum amount of Percocet that I can get by with each day to mitigate the back pain until we figure out next steps. The cancer has pushed through my vertebrae and created compression fractures in my spine.

There is a minimally invasive procedure called vertebroplasty, as well as a similar procedure called a "kyphoplasty, that many swear by. Perhaps that is in my very near future. I hope something is.

Coincidentally, today is a comparatively good day. The sun is shining and it is pushing 70 degrees in the Greater Cincinnati area. I was able to get outside and clean the yard up a bit (I will get in trouble with Diana for that when she gets home). Today is the best I have felt in weeks. Spring has sprung.

Next steps are to head back to MD Anderson to consult with my medical oncologist there. While there, we will do a PSMA PET scan (my seventh!) to see what can be seen in my soft tissue. The recent MRIs have been able to see the cancer that has metastasized to bone, but there has to be something else going on.

Despite it all, my PSA is rising again and rising quickly. A biomarker that typically chugs along at a glacial pace, if at all, is now doing this:

3/04/2024   16.2
3/06/2024   18.3
3/12/2024   22.8
3/19/2024   25.1

Something evil is going on inside despite everyone's best efforts and the PSMA PET scan will find it. I have cycled through pretty much all FDA-approved treatments for metastatic, castrate-resistant prostate cancer with moderate success. Nothing is really working now.

The most likely next step is an immunotherapy clinical trial, but there are parameters that need to be met before that is an option. Depending on the trial chosen, one's PSA has to be below 50 ng/dl and at the rate things are going, I am not hopeful I will slide in under that wire a month from now.

I've previously written about a Hobson's Choice, which is an apparently free decision when there is no real alternative. I may soon face one of these again, which is the possibility of having to start back on chemotherapy to get my PSA down far enough so that I can gain entry into a Phase I, immuno-therapy-based clinical trial. In a Phase I clinical trial, efficacy data is early at best and the maximum safe dose is not yet known, and the attempts to calibrate that may result in serious adverse events, including the possibility of the really bad serious adverse event that I won't mention here. Ugh.

But all of that said, while in Houston we are going to go to a Houston Astros baseball game at Minute Maid Park and see our friends Roz and Alan Pactor, great supporters and sister and brother- in-law of my dear friend, Steve Tyrell.

Life goes on — gotta enjoy it while you can.

STEVE ABBOTT

BUCKET LISTS

THE lyrics from Kenny Chesney's song "Bucket" still make me laugh every time I hear them... "I made a bucket list, changed the B to an F, I gave my give a damn the finger, so it got up and left." One of the liberties you can give yourself when you are not sure how much time you have left (none of us do, in fact) is the freedom to go wherever you want, anywhere in the world, throwing caution to the wind and not really caring what it costs. For most people, it's probably never really that simple.

Either there is nothing imminent to indicate your demise, so therefore budget is still an issue. Or there is something making you think your time is limited and if so, you likely don't feel well enough at that point to jet set around the world with no restrictions or practical limitations. That's where I find myself these days. There are places I wish I could have gotten to that I likely never will, and that's ok.

I will likely never fully get the images of thatched, over-the-water bungalows in Tahiti or Bora Bora that I have seen in travel magazines out of my head. I never got the chance to go visit my friend Gerry during the many years that he lived in New Zealand, which would of course have led to a side jaunt to Australia. My friend Marco has invited us to join them on visits to South Africa, and that is not likely to happen now as well. The Maldives, Iceland, the Canary Islands, Patagonia, Portugal, Germany, the Argentinian wine country... I could go on and on, and the truth of the matter is that it makes my back hurt to think of making an overnight, round-trip flight in an uncomfortable airline seat to get to any of those places.

But when I think of the places I have gone, I am overwhelmed. I grew up in Latonia, Kentucky. My parents did not have college educations, and upward mobility was a hard thing to achieve without that all- important degree (there were no TikTok millionaire options back then). My father was a blue-collar worker, and my mother was a stay-at-home mom. Financial resources were limited and travel — a purely discretionary item - was one of the last things on the list. And yet, it was a priority for our family and my parents somehow made it work. We always managed to get away as a family and those are some of the greatest memories of my life (your mind somehow conveniently manages to block out the memories of the incessant squabbling amongst pre-teens in the back of a station wagon on a 16-hour drive from Latonia, Kentucky to Palm Beach, Florida).

I could have never dreamed at the time, nor would I have dared to dream, that I would get to visit islands throughout the Caribbean, destinations sites in

Europe, multiple visits to the Canadian Rockies, plus multiple trips to Hawaii, Mexico, and most U.S. states. I have been to Napa Valley more than twenty times. We visited my friend Bruce in southern California more than 25 times. I have been to Italy 26 times. 26 times! Most people will be lucky to go there once in their lifetime.

While there are still so many places I would like to go, I am content to think back on those many adventures and focus on what is now achievable and reasonable. Even practical considerations come to mind... what if something goes wrong while there? How would I pay for health care since my insurance would not be accepted? And can I trust that the quality of care delivered will be sufficient until I can get back home?

It is now the end of March 2024. Despite the chaos of the past few weeks, the gods have seen fit to open up a window at the end of this week where we can go to Tampa, Florida to attend the wine-soaked "Cheers for Charity" fund-raiser put on by our dear friends Ron & Tami. This is an amazing event held at their house each year that raises hundreds of thousands of dollars for children's charities in the Greater Tampa area. We've never been able to attend before. While there, we will have dinner at the iconic Bern's Steak House which will be our first time there. It is legendary — they have more than half a million bottles of wine, for God's sake!

We will rent a convertible and drive to Key West at our own pace. I have never been able to make that amazing, 100+ mile drive out over the open ocean from Miami to Key West. I have never been to Key West. There is going to be a solar eclipse while we are there. It is going to be an amazing trip and I feel up to doing it.

I am hopeful that we will be able to make the 40th anniversary trip to France and Monaco in June, but I am being realistic about that and not count-ing on it. I am also not ready to turn it loose because my brother and sister-in-law are planning on joining us for that trip. Later in the summer, we are going to make a multi- day, chauffeured trip throughout Kentucky to enjoy my home state's "Bourbon Country" with four sets of dear friends. It's early but that feels very "doable." It's still very much on the list.

There is a common denominator here. My thoughts now turn more to making trips that allow me to see friends and spend time with people I care about rather than checking a box. I have never had much interest in visiting all fifty U.S. states. It feels more like a collection to me, and I am not much of a collector of anything other than good wine.. There are way too many amazing things still on the list to ever get to, and that would be the case even if I lived to be a hundred years old.

An occasional trip to Lexington to see my father. A day trip to my brother's lake house. An overnight bourbon tasting trip with my mom to Louisville or Bardstown. Perhaps a trip to New Orleans with Diana (she has always wanted to go but has never been there before). Bunt singles and the occasional double rather than swinging for the fences. And that's ok.

PLAY BALL!

THIS chapter is dedicated to my paternal grandfather, Merrill Abbott.

The "boys of summer" are back. There is something very assuring about traditions —the same things happen, year in and year out — especially when they are beloved like baseball in America.

I absolutely LOVED baseball as a young child. I (barely) played for the Covington Firefighters, the feared local dynasty in "knothole" baseball. It may not surprise you that like many millions of other 12-year-olds at any given time in America, I knew I was going to be a professional baseball player when I grew up, notwithstanding the annual struggle to make the cut and be on the team (it was always dicey).

The Covington Firefighters could afford to be choosy. There were years when the team was the most feared group of 100-pound, 12-year-old baseball players in the city. Being a second-string shortstop or utility infielder was good enough, as long as I could wear that red-and-white cotton uniform with a big "C" on the front. Our coach — Lou Brockhoff — was a legend in his own mind who thought nothing of humiliating little kids in pursuit of toughening them up (a certain episode of him making me run the bases repeatedly in front of my teammates chanting "I'm afraid of the ball" after lifting my head on a grounder and letting it go through my legs into the outfield comes to mind). Oh, the stuff I would not put up with any more in my life.

In the mid-1970's, was there any kid in Greater Cincinnati who **didn't** want to be a professional baseball player someday? Within walking distance of the diamond at Glenn O. Swing Elementary school was Cincinnati's Riverfront Stadium, home of one of the greatest teams in baseball history — Cincinnati's "Big Red Machine." What began with a fateful trade of Lee May to the Houston Astros for Joe Morgan after the end of the 1971 season quickly led to a "Murderer's Row" lineup of Pete Rose, Johnny Bench, Joe Morgan, Tony Perez, George Foster, and others. Even Dave Concepcion and Cesar Geronimo, who came to the Reds as players who could barely eke out a .200 batting average, became reliable, near .300 hitters, batting seventh or eighth in the lineup. There was no rest for opposing pitchers when facing the Big Red Machine.

For a 12-year-old baseball fan from Covington, Kentucky, it was a dream to be able to go to the "big city" of Cincinnati for a Reds game. My parents worked hard, so the opportunities to go with my parents were limited (although I am happy to say that our entire family was in the stands the night of my 39th birthday, when Pete Rose notched hit #4,192 to surpass Ty Cobb).

My grandfather — Merrill Abbott — would occasionally take me to a game. Looking back on it, it was hard for him to do that. He was not well. Among other maladies, he had emphysema and struggled to breathe. I remember the thrill of going to a Reds game being somewhat tempered by what a physical ordeal it was for him. Every step was a struggle for him and there were no "handicapped accessible" seats back then. Ascending the steps into the nosebleed seats was a struggle. Take two steps and wait. Take another two steps and wait for Grandpa. I didn't really understand it at the time, but I look back on it now and realize what a sacrifice it was for him to take me to do it. Of course, I had my ball glove with me (necessary equipment to catch a foul ball in the stands) and I was raring to go — ready to run all the way from the parking lot to watch batting practice.

Over the years, I have lost my zeal for baseball. My previously mentioned attention span disorder makes it hard for me to devote three hours to a game, 162 times a year. I find myself more drawn to it this season due to nostalgia and may find myself back in the ballpark more often. Traditions suddenly feel a bit more important.

ACCIDENTAL BRILLIANCE

THIS chapter could just as easily be titled, "sometimes it's better to be lucky than good" — a variation on the quote often attributed to 1930's-era Hall-of-Fame baseball pitcher Lefty Gomez. Looking back over this manuscript (it feels cool to say that), it occurs to me that there was something monumental in our married life that has taken place in the last year that I haven't mentioned until now...we moved.

Sitting across the aisle from each other on a plane, Diana buckled in, put her headset on, and got ready to watch whatever movie it was she was going to watch. Me — ever the fiddler — opened my briefcase and brought out a mass of paper(s) to read, rip up and throw away. Lighten the load... get a few things off the list. Really important things were transferred onto an index card to make sure that the rolling to-do list stays updated and relevant. No rest for the wicked.

About an hour into the flight, two things happened: (1) I felt tired and (2) my thoughts turned to moving. The post-pandemic real estate market in the summer of 2023 in the greater Cincinnati area was white-hot, with housing inventory being so tight that people were getting above asking price and selling on listing day with no inspections and — if you were lucky enough to hit the trifecta — the previously elusive cash deal.

For the rest of the six-hour flight, I ran through scenarios in my head. The easiest thing — by far — was to stay where we were — a lovely four-bedroom house in Edgewood, Kentucky with a backyard oasis that few people in an under-30% federal tax bracket were lucky enough to enjoy. We had lived there for over 25 years and our "stuff" sprawled throughout three floors, whether we needed it to or not. After all, you take up as much room as you have. The clincher though was that we were one of the lucky ones... we had a mortgage locked in at 2.875% - a rate so low that I never felt the need to pay the remaining mortgage down because we could earn more than that by investing it.

Yet, I couldn't stop thinking about the fact that maybe the time to move was now. I felt good at the time, with my PSA hovering in the low teens (a luxury for me). The thing I kept coming back to was WITH advanced prostate cancer... the road does not get easier. The idea of trying to pack up three floors worth of stuff, accumulated over almost 30 years, at some time in the future when I am not doing as well, suddenly had my undivided attention.

Later that evening, out of the blue, I asked Diana, "what would you think about the possibility of us moving?" One stark difference between Diana and I — and one that I am sure characterizes lots of married couples — is that Diana is constantly researching and shopping. She shops whether she is going to buy things or not. I acquire things when needed. Shopping when I am not going to buy seems like a waste of time, so I get what I need when I need it (although "need" is a very subjective thing).

Diana had been looking at houses off and on for years. She would occasionally show homes to me, and I would give it my cursory, what she calls, "man look." So, once I mentioned the possibility of us moving, she was ready to roll. By the time we left the island a week later, we had decided to move and had already set two goals: (1) find our new home and move in by July 1 and (2) then and only then, get our house ready to sell and list it by August 1. If we were going to do this, I did not want to be stuck if the house sold quickly (a good problem) but we then had to move to an apartment, then move again once we bought the next house.

I found a house online that I loved. A two-bedroom ranch was the right size for us. The thought of not climbing three flights of stairs multiple times a day was very appealing. Two days after we returned home from vacation, we toured the first of two houses with our realtor friend Julie Feagan. We fell in love immediately, so much so that we debated whether to even see the second house. We had found what we wanted on the first shot. Our offer was accepted, financing was pre-approved. We closed on the new home and moved in on July 1, literally right on schedule.

We charged forward at a furious pace, packing up boxes, taking things to Goodwill, throwing things out, painting, repairing, buffing hardwood floors, and eating carry-out food pretty much every night at the old house. Remarkably, and with no forced engineering to meet an arbitrary date, we listed the house on the morning of August 1 — the EXACT date that we originally set as our goal. We had more than 20 showings that day with 16 bona fide offers. That evening, with nervous anticipation, we accepted a cash offer, way above the asking price, with no inspections and closing in a week. A week? Seriously? Lo and behold, we closed on the evening of August 8. The whole process was nothing short of miraculous.

Seven short weeks later, I woke up with such excruciating back pain that I could not get out of bed. It was the date of our annual Cincinnati Cancer Advisors "ASCO Direct Best of Oncology" symposium, a thought leadership event for oncology professionals. It's a big deal, and obligations are obligations, so I struggled to try to make it there that day to assist my colleagues. I couldn't answer the bell. I was in so much back pain that it literally hurt to breathe. What we learned later was that the cancer had metastasized to my spine.

I am very selective about things that I think are the result of divine intervention. That is a pretty high bar in my judgment. But I am left to wonder… what caused me on May 11, 2023, to begin thinking about moving when in fact, it did not seem to be imperative to do so at the time? Something caused me to think that it might make sense to do that now, even though it made no financial sense. How would I explain this to my dear friend and financial advisor, Paul McCauley (who, as it turned out, was a big supporter of the idea)?

At the risk of overstating the case, it is nothing short of a miracle that we moved when we did…and that things came together the way they did. As a bonus, we could not love our new house any more than we do.

Sometimes, it's better to be lucky than good.

STATE OF NOTHINGNESS

THIS chapter is dedicated to David & Ginny Wayland, Lew & Judy Clements, Ted & Mary Ann Weiss, Henry & Gayle Wells and Cliff & Kathy Daly, who, along with my parents, were kind enough to indulge me as a 13-year know-it-all while a member at Trinity Episcopal Church in Covington, Kentucky.

Once someone with a life- threatening illness moves beyond the whistling-past-the-graveyard stage (see chapter 34), I think it's natural to start getting your affairs in order. For most people, that's a blend of financial and spiritual affairs. Just to make sure that I am leaving things as well organized as possible for Diana, I have begun the financial part.

Getting my spiritual house in order is a bit of a different thing. To be honest, I don't really "practice" religion anymore (for a special treat, find the video online of former NBA superstar Allen Iverson talking about practice — it is hilarious). Thankfully, I have enough verbal/muscle memory from years spent reciting the same liturgy over and over that I could probably return to church today and never miss a beat.

I was raised Christian as a member of the Episcopal Church — the American equivalent of the U.K's Anglican Church. I lovingly describe the Episcopal Church as "Catholic without all the rules and guilt." Introduced to the Episcopal Church by my parents somewhere around the age of 11 or 12, soon thereafter, I was baptized and confirmed by a Bishop in a somewhat bewildering ceremony that concluded with congratulations from other parishioners and a post-service celebration involving cake and punch.

As my parents were the adult leaders of the church youth group, what I believe to be full-blown nepotism resulted in me being a quickly elected President of the youth group. One major perk of the gig was that I was sponsored by the parish to attend a national youth conference at the YMCA Camp of the Rockies in Estes Park, Colorado. I attended with my fellow officers: Brad Fry and Dottie Clements. We were under the watchful eye of our chaperone, Lew Clements, an affable, good-natured, well- humored, high school music teacher and band leader who had the perfect temperament for the trip. He was always patient with a wry smile and thoughtful gaze that instilled confidence. This was my first flight on an airplane so the whole experience was nothing short of intoxicating.

I will never forget the opening session of the youth conference. There were literally hundreds — many hundreds — of other kids from around the country in attendance with their chaperones/sponsors. Andre Crouch, a well-known gospel singer performed, then a stand-up comedy performance from Mike

Warnke (for just as much fun as the Allen Iverson video, Google "Christian comedian Mike Warnke" and check out this guy's Wikipedia page — as it turns out, he had no business being in front of a group of barely teenage kids). That said, I will never forget one of the guy's jokes. He was talking about different religions and in describing Buddhism, referred to nirvana as a "state of nothingness," which he quickly followed up by saying "I thought that was Iowa." Killer stuff for a crowd of 13-year-olds.

The handful of years following that conference was when I peaked as a practicing Christian. By the time I married in the Episcopal Church at the ripe old age of 21, I could recite the liturgy from memory, word-for-word. With my attention span already starting to wane, sermons seemed ever longer and — if I am honest — I began to think of church as a perfectly good way to waste a Sunday morning.

During those formative years, and with my exalted position as youth group President, I was honored to become part of my parents' inner circle of fellow church goers — the Waylands, Dalys, Weisses, Clements, and Wells. They were some of the "movers and shakers" of Trinity Episcopal Church, who often spent time at our house with my parents in a post-movie discussion, a coffee-and-dessert gathering after a play at Cincinnati's Playhouse in the Park, or to discuss whatever book was currently ascending the *New York Times* best-seller list. Real egghead stuff to a 13 year old.

As such, they were sitting ducks for my witty repartee consisting of baseball trivia and whatever other insightful comments that my barely teenage brain could come up with at the time *(during this era, my father would also call me a "Philadelphia Lawyer." Because this was pre-Google, I had no idea what that meant, but I could tell he didn't mean it as a compliment given that he was generally exasperated and would call me that through slightly clenched teeth. As it turns out, it was a backhanded compliment!).*

My father tolerated it to a certain point, but ultimately dismissed me to bed as I had overstayed my welcome and, in his estimation, worn everyone out. This group included some of the most gracious people I have ever met and who to this day still hold a special place in my heart. They did not wear their religion on their sleeves. Like so many Episcopalians, they were very understated in their evangelism (or lack thereof) and in a weird sort of way, they practiced but they did not preach. In many ways, they were the model for how I do things in my own life. I am very much a "Golden Rule" guy. The Golden Rule makes things incredibly simple and when followed, removes the barriers that divide people along religious lines while making the world a better place.

Lately, I have found myself thinking more often about what happens when the end comes. Logic can sometimes get in the way of faith for me, and I wonder whether we do just pass on to some "state of nothingness" (like Iowa) or even just cease to exist. I think back to March 2000, on the bottom part of the ski mountain at stunning Lake Louise in Banff National Park in Alberta, Canada. As I often did, I skied ahead of Diana, going as fast as I could (as Diana would call it, "hair on fire"). While looking up the mountain and waiting for her to come down in her careful, hourglass-shaped twists and turns, some dude slammed into me doing whatever-the-maximum-speed-that-someone-can-ski speed.

I woke to the aroma of smelling salts, with a group of ski patrollers standing around me, in a fairly large puddle of my own blood, which was pouring out of my nose at the time. I remember bright sunshine in my eyes and one of the ski patrollers asking me where I was from, and "who is the President of the United States?" to which I answered "Bill Clinton." My eye socket was broken, along with my wrist and one of my thumbs. I have no memory of what happened, the assailant-on-skis did not stick around to help, and there was no video to shed any light on how it all transpired. It was awful, but at least I was alive.

In the aftermath of that accident, I have thought many times about the fact that that could have been it. The end. Game over. If the impact had been greater, or the blunt force applied at a different place on my head, I could have been dead just as easily as if I was knocked unconscious. And if so, was that it? No gentle, comforting, white light, or peaceful tunnel to pass through, no paved streets of gold if you had been good, or bubbling cauldrons of hell fire if you had been bad? Just... gone... over... a state of nothingness. I have had similar thoughts following surgery where anesthesia was administered and you just go off to sleep, where you felt nothing, and remembered nothing — as if nothing ever happened. Just lights out.

It's almost fifty years later and I must confess that my church attendance is dismal. My spirituality is more humanist in nature — informed by science, inspired by art, and motivated by compassion. Will I go through a reckoning prior to passing someday, or will I just continue to practice the Golden Rule, be nice to people, and take my chances? Too early to know.

My head tells me that there may be no bright light or tunnel to pass through —maybe the afterlife is just a state of nothingness. However, my heart tells me that there is something spectacular that defies explanation that created this universe that transcends all our understanding. Perhaps there is something to go on to after all, in whatever form that may be. The truth is that none of us really know, but I am happy in the knowledge that my faith and practices were formed and informed by observing the quiet grace and kindness of people like those mentors at Trinity Episcopal Church, whose attention and approval I coveted at the age of 13.

MY MUSE —
DIANA MARIE (SEWELL) ABBOTT

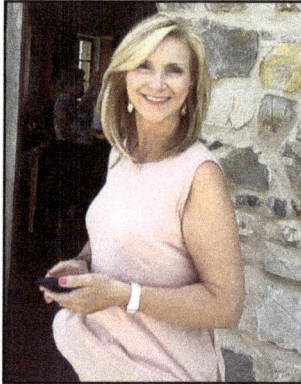

*This is one of my favorite photos of Diana. Shortly after this photo was taken,
I accepted a job as the Chief Financial Officer of Montèverdi Tuscany.*

NOW that I am a "writer," I can have a "muse" and my muse is Diana Marie Abbott (nee Sewell). In ancient Greek religion and mythology, the Muses are the inspirational goddesses of literature, science, and the arts. My muse is the person who gives me the ideas and the desire to create.

This feels appropriate in so many ways. Those that know Diana know that she is a fan of science fiction, the supernatural, and the ethereal (and dare I say, the occult?). In fact, it was she who first told me (jokingly) many, many years ago, that she was named for Diana... Artemis — the goddess of the hunt and in Greek mythology — the goddess of domestic animals. I vouch without hesitation that she is the goddess of our three domestic animals: Toby, Ellie and Coco.

It is also appropriate because she truly has been my muse — encouraging me to begin writing over 25 years ago, even to the point of suggesting that I pursue it as a career. I never viewed that as an option for a variety of reasons but she has never stopped encouraging me to give it a try.

I first saw her in 1977, in Mr. Gamble's ninth grade algebra class at Holmes High School in Covington, Kentucky. The class probably had 30 to 35 students. She sat far enough away from me that I didn't interact with her. Because I was too shy to go out of my way to introduce myself, we went through the entire semester without even sayiing "Hello" to one another. My sophomore year came and went, and as I wasn't in any of her classes, and our interactions were limited to passing each other in the hallway between "bells" (Holmes had close to 3,000 students in total, across grades 7-12, and is spread out across a large campus, so there weren't many opportunities for socializing while marching on to the next class).

Ahhh, but our junior year! When I returned from summer break, Diana was seated directly behind me in homeroom. I don't even know if schools still have homerooms, but at the time, it was this slightly odd arrangement where you and selected classmates started the school day. Not wildly dissimilar to roll call in the military, we'd gather, recite the Pledge of Allegiance, listen to announcements, kill a bit of time, then head out for your first class when the first bell rang.

I was so smitten with Diana that I did what pretty much any sixteen-year-old going on eight-years-old would do, which was make jokes and random observations that she did not find amusing at the time. She had gorgeous, long brown hair and thanks to my endless pestering, she mastered the eye roll at a fairly young age.

I acted like a fool throughout the school year without ever asking her out (whatever that means when you're a teenager). During the summer break, one of my buddies — who knew that I was crazy about her — finally baited me into mustering up the courage to go to her house and ask her out. His logic was "you'll never know if you don't ask" and "what is the worst thing she can do?" (to which I said... "uhh, Carl - have you ever heard of rejection?").

I was a nervous wreck as he drove me to her house. Of course, she answered the door, so I made some inane, awkward conversation, then finally just came right out with it, fully expecting her to say "no." She said "yes," and I was absolutely dumbfounded. We made a date for the following Friday night...

....and we have been inseparable since that day for the last 45 years.

We often say that we not only grew up together, but that we have done everything together. There is one big exception... we never had children. Over the years, many people have asked us why we did not have children. For me, this was never an easy decision, but the answer from my perspective is one that might cause the reader to now roll your eyes. Diana was, and always has been, so perfect for me that I never wanted to change what we had or risk our relationship in any way. My concern about raising children bringing too much pressure to bear on a relationship, even fearing that this stress could result in our marriage not lasting (we've all seen it happen before). I don't think Diana ever worried about that to the degree that I did. Moreso, if either of us had pushed to have children, I suspect the other would have readily and happily agreed and it would have been great.

We have often said that we have done everything together, and we have. "Peas and carrots," as Forrest Gump would say. Some people have mistakenly assumed that we did not have children because we wanted to selfishly pursue a life of travel, fancy dinners out, nice cars and the like.

If that was the case, we would have never dedicated ourselves to taking in (now) eight rescue dogs over the years. We've had "fear biters," dogs with separation anxiety, puppy-mill-abuse cases, unsocialized, untrained, and not-house-trained dogs over the last 30 years. We have taken in misfit dogs and trained them into sweet and loyal companions. We have turned down dinners so we can get home and feed them and "not leave them too long". We have even, when necessary, taken separate vacations so that the dogs never had to go to the kennel. We have spent thousands of dollars caring for them, and we have tearfully and jointly made the final, hard decision to say goodbye to our beloved dogs — five times. I know that we would have managed children just fine and ironically enough, we are now 61 years old and still not "empty nesters" thanks to our dogs.

When I say we have pretty much done everything together, that also extends to cancer. Diana was diagnosed with triple-negative breast cancer in January 2015 at the age of 52, just sixteen months after I began treatment for my own cancer. Although I knew by then that my case was incurable, I was nonetheless physically recovered from the surgery and salvage radiation so I was feeling good from a physical perspective. Her diagnosis was devastating to me as, quite honestly, I would much rather "go first" than spend one day without her.

Her treatment regimen was brutal, beginning with the dreaded ACT chemo cocktail — Adriamycin, Cytoxin and Taxol — followed by radiation and a lumpectomy to remove any trace of the cancer. I watched her turn various shades of gray, lose her hair, eyebrows, fingernails, and toenails, but she never lost her sense of humor. She used it as an opportunity to purchase about two dozen wigs and went to work each day as a different "personality" — sometimes as a blonde, other days as a redhead, some days with short hair, and other days with long hair. Hats were optional and she wore them often. Although I know she did not feel well enough to do it, she went on our trip with six friends during chemo because she did not want to disappoint anyone.

Diana was and is a warrior. The only time I saw her cry during chemo was when she developed shingles, which found it's way in after chemotherapy took her immune system down. She was in so... much... pain, and I felt so **** helpless. I am happy to report that nine years later, her scans are clean, and she is showing no evidence of disease.

We also work together — successfully, I might add — at Cincinnati Cancer Advisors. We are very blessed.

When I say that we have gone through pretty much everything together, I mean everything. A good number of men (most, in fact) with advanced prostate cancer will go through "male menopause" due to the androgen deprivation therapy used to control the pace of the disease progression and mitigate its spread. Trust me... a marriage has not been truly tested until (a) you've worked together at the same company in a direct reporting relationship (I get to wear the pants at work, but trust me, I am very careful about that) and (b) both partners are going through menopause... again, at the same time.

It is a cliché for sure, but she is my rock. My everything in life. My "ride or die." My muse.

WHAT MIGHT HAVE BEEN

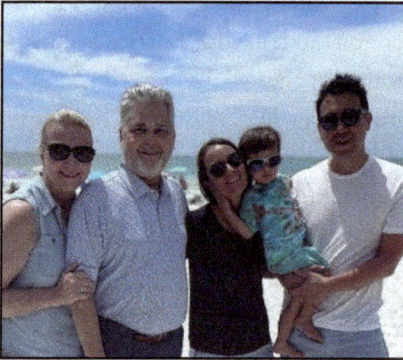

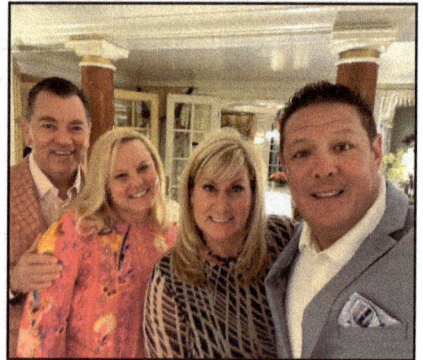

Left: *Diana Abbott, Steve Abbott, Lauren Amorico, Leonardo "Leo" Amorico and Marco Amorico at Anna Maria Island, Florida. Another gathering of our friend.* Right: *Ron Broadrick, Tami Broadrick, Donna Candiotti and Mike Herrera. Whenever we gather with these kind folks, two things are guaranteed to be the case: fancy blazers and some worthy charity will benefit.*

WOW, what a week! Thanks to a break between treatments, my wish for a five-day holiday in Florida came true. My back was still killing me (I hope to be able to report a successful procedure to alleviate that pain soon) but, thankfully, Diana proved herself to be an amazing luggage lugger who would not let me pick up, carry, or even think about moving my overstuffed suitcases.

We began our adventure in Tampa where we attended the aforementioned "Cheers for Charity" fundraiser, hosted by our dear friends Ron and Tami Broadrick. A wonderful surprise was attending the Friday night celebration at Bern's Steakhouse, a pre-event filled with fantastic friends, food, and wines.

The Saturday event was truly an amazing and inspirational event, taking place at a sprawling, table-for-100 people ... in their driveway. We were in awe at seeing paddles raised repeatedly in support of underprivileged children with incredibly generous donations. This intimate event raised $1.4 million for a host of children's charities throughout Florida.

Over the past eight years, Ron and Tami have raised approximately $7 million for children's charities throughout Florida. I find what they do to be especially compelling given that they do not have children of their own, yet they dedicate a significant amount of their time and effort to these various children's causes. To learn more about the Broadrick Family Foundation, or to donate, please visit https://www.broadrickfamilyfoundation.org/home.

We were also very fortunate to meet up with our dear friends Marco and Lauren Amorico and their precious son Leonardo (Leo) as the trio had arrived from Italy to Anna Maria Island the night before. Honestly, I had been worried that I might never see them again given the state of my health and the difficulty of traveling long distances. But *ecco qui!* — they magically ended up in the Florida Keys, arriving just in time for us to be able to spend time with them. We all had a wonderful lunch right on the beach on a beautiful afternoon with our toes in the sand. I couldn't believe how well things lined up.

As we were returning from dinner in Tampa on Friday night, something caused me to think back to another seminal moment during my early teens. I have written about my family's annual vacation to somewhere/anywhere in Florida. My father had fallen in love with the Sunshine State and as a meter reader for Cincinnati Gas & Electric, he had followed up on an opportunity to potentially relocate and take a similar job with Tampa Gas & Electric.

One day, while performing one of my weekly chores of emptying the wastebasket in his office (basically, a desk, chair and bookshelf that adjoined my parent's bedroom), I stumbled onto a piece of black "carbon paper." Only people of a certain age will remember carbon paper, but at the risk of oversimplifying, it's how people made copies back in the 1970s. It was a flimsy, black sheet that was placed between the page being written and the copy that was created by the carbon. I remember holding it up to the light and seeing my father's flowy, cursive writing, his perfect penmanship expressing his interest in a job at TG&E.

I was horrified, notwithstanding the fact that I had no business reading his letter in the first place. As much as I loved going to Florida with my family, I was a soon-to-be-teenager in Northern Kentucky and I simply did not want to move. I recall pulling the family fire alarm and creating a bunch of drama around it, which complicated my father's process.

As it turns out, it was a moot point. My father had undergone back surgery, which at that les enlightened time disqualified him from the job. But what hit me while Diana and I were in Tampa was... what if he had somehow landed the job and moved our family to Florida? His disqualification was due to the comparatively primitive state of orthopedic surgery at the time and the fact that employers were able to delve into your personal health details as part of their evaluation.

Logic tells me that nothing that transpired over the weekend would have ever happened if my father had moved us to Tampa. For starters, I wouldn't have met Diana, ipso facto, I would not have spent the last 45 years with her. I originally met Ron and Tami Broadrick at a gathering of the Lexington Cancer Foundation, at an event where I was representing Monteverdi Tuscany, a job I never would have had if our family had moved to Tampa.

I also met Marco Amorico through my affiliation with Monteverdi Tuscany on one of my work trips to Italy. Marco's family are the owners of Access Italy, a renowned destination management company in Italy, which is what originally connected us (and I highly recommend them for any trips to Italy). From that initial contact, Marco and I became instant friends. Nearly every visit thereafter included a meet-up where Marco and I drank great Italian wines, accompanied by Cacio e Pepe or Pasta Amatriciana. Diana and I went to Marco and Lauren's wedding on the beach in Anna Maria Island, Florida — right where we were able to reconnect with them during this trip.

My head was suddenly spinning as I thought about it all. Nothing... literally NOTHING... about this trip would have happened if my father had changed jobs nearly 50 years ago. In discussing this with my father and brother upon our return, my brother added that he would have never met his wife of 32 years if we had moved. My sisters would surely not have met their spouses either. And I certainly would not have been in the job I am in now, which turns out to be the most meaningful work I have ever done in my life.

We all have these "Butterfly Effect" moments in our lives, where one thing that happened differently would have changed our life forever, and in a profound way. It is humbling to think that virtually everything that I love about my life today would have been different if a single event - which was more central to my father and what he wanted to do with his life — had taken place.

So I asked my father at lunch whether he would have taken the job if it had been offered. He thought about it for a minute, then said that he didn't know. That as great as it sounded to move to Florida at the time, he doesn't know if he would have actually pulled the trigger. I really like Tampa, but thank goodness that things turned out the way they did. Who knows what might have been, but I know that things would not have turned out as well for me as they did if we had made that move.

RENT THE CONVERTIBLE.
USE THE MILES. WIN EVERY DAY.

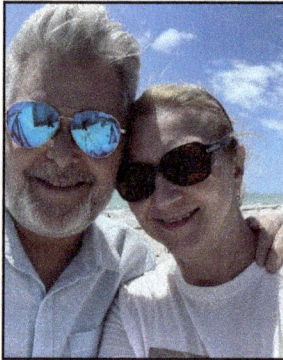

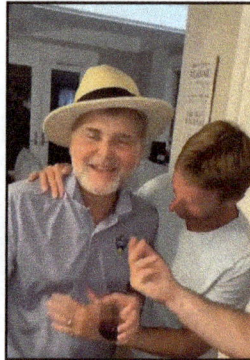

Left: *Steve and Diana on the drive from Tampa, Florida to Key West, Florida. I have wanted to make this drive for decades — a recent break from treatment gave me the opportunity to finally make it happen.* Right: *Ron Broadrick, Tami Broadrick, Donna Candiotti and Mike Herrera. Whenever we guSteve enduring harassment from his dear friend Mike Grubbs. This is one of many barely memorable events that led to the creation of "Team 47."*

SURVIVE *and* ADVANCE

THIS chapter is dedicated to my dear friends Traci and Todd Gruenwald and Mike and Jenni Grubbs. Like so many other chance meetings in life, I met the Grubbs at Traci's annual Christmas party, where I was introduced to everyone gathered there by a slightly overserved Traci as "my good friend, Steve". The crowd had a great time with that and for many years after, I was known by that group as "Traci's good friend, Steve." Fast forward almost 15 years later to a beach house in Santa Rosa Beach where Traci, Todd, Mike, Jenni, Diana, and I were awash in some sort of bourbon-laced concoction that we somehow ended up naming the "47." The 47 now lives in infamy within our friendship...and has taken on other meanings, none of which make any sense to any of us and is generally used by the males in some sort of juvenile fashion. None of us really remember how "the 47" came about but the main thing I remember is that I ended up wearing a fedora for most of the evening. I have fun every time I am near these people.

I am still on a high from the Florida adventure. For many, many years, I had wanted to drive the Florida Keys from start to finish, partly because I knew it would evoke thoughts of a lifestyle feted in the songs of Jimmy Buffett and Kenny Chesney.

Ironically, I was never the type who would "chuck it all" and move to the Keys or the Caribbean, believing that everything would just work out. But having the pluck to do something like that now was something that I aspired to.

One thing that I am thankful about with respect to having cancer is that it has allowed me to do things I might not have ever done otherwise, and I am the better for it. Now, don't let all this cavalier talk fool you into thinking that I am the type of guy that rents convertibles on vacation. Considering the many trips we have taken in our lives, I can count on one hand the number of times that I ponied up the extra money to rent the convertible. It just always seemed like so much more money and I figured that I could always just roll the windows down.

But not this trip. No, this was a rent-the-convertible trip if there ever was one. We easily spent double on the candy-apple red Ford Mustang rather than a Nissan Altima or Toyota Corolla, but it was worth every cent. I am pretty sure I grinned ear-to-ear all the way from Key Largo to Key West. Definitely rent the convertible.

The resort where we stayed in Key Largo was just supposed to be for one night, but we loved it too much to leave so quickly. I booked a second night there at a price I would have normally recoiled at...and I felt great about it. We loved our extra time there. No regrets.

STEVE ABBOTT

After all, the following week I was supposed to fly back to Houston at the crack-of-ridiculous on a Monday morning for a full week of scans and tests, but the schedule changed. Shoulda', coulda' change my flight and hotel arrangements to allow me to be here the extra day with Diana and my dogs? The money it would cost to make the changes felt prohibitive, but I do have airline miles and hotel points. It still hurts to use so many but what else are they for? Using them bought me a full extra day here with the people I love most. Use the miles.

One of my best friends called me to check on me the other day. He is a fellow cancer warrior who was diagnosed with the "other good cancer to have" — thyroid cancer — as a very young man. I use quotes in the preceding sentence because people often discount prostate cancer and thyroid cancer as somehow the best cancers. Jeff and I both have battle scars (literally) to show for a lengthy battle with cancer, and his counsel and his words meant the world to me.

As we were about to hang up the phone, he said something to me that I am likely to never forget: "You have to win every day." It occurs to me that the simple acts above are "wins." I did what I wanted to do, no longer so concerned about what it cost. Today was a win because I did not have to leave, and I am enjoying a beautiful late spring day with my patio door open because of it. No regrets. Win every day.

Jeff's words also remind me of something else that brings this chapter full circle. Another dear friend — Mike Grubbs, mentioned above — who I met by chance at a Christmas party oh-so-many years ago — made a very courageous choice because of a medical condition that is slowly but surely robbing him of his sight. He was also diagnosed with a life-changing condition as a very young man, and I remember him telling me that he sold his business and moved his family to Florida a few years ago because he wanted to spend every day with them and see beauty in every direction for as long as he could see it. Simply put, he made the choice to win every day, and he inspires me as well.

My new goal is to figure out what a win looks like each day and do my best to make it happen. There will be days ahead when just staying alive is a win. But hopefully, a successful cancer treatment awaits. Fingers crossed that there will be a procedure that can relieve the incredible back pain that I have been experiencing for the past six months. If those things happen, you can be certain that my definition of a "win" will change, and you will see me touching all the bases. I just need to make sure I have enough money, airline miles and hotel points left over so that I can always rent the convertible.

THE MONKEY DIED

THIS chapter is dedicated to Sophia Kappen and Will Kays, both of whom lost their cancer battle way too early while participating in a clinical trial that they hoped would save their lives.

Time for an update on where things stand. In March 2024, I underwent a hurriedly arranged surgery to place two renal stents. This procedure was necessary due to a rapid decline in kidney function due to scar tissue that had formed in both ureters from past radiation to my pelvis and abdomen. The adjustment to the stents has been relatively problem-free, except for the bleeding that resulted from irritation to the ureters from the stents themselves and the need to be on a blood thinner to avoid development of blood clots, or at least manage them when they occur.

I read recently that cancer patients, on average, are nine times more likely to develop blood clots than people without cancer. Nine times! I am certainly not qualified to comment on why that is the case, and quite honestly, most of the medical professionals who I have asked are somewhat hard-pressed to explain it as well. I guess we can just leave it at...for some reason, cancer patients have "stickier" blood after developing cancer.

As noted above, I've lost a notable amount of blood into my urine which has caused low red blood counts and a degree of anemia. Because there are events coming in my near-term future that will be complicated by being on a blood thinner, I underwent a procedure this past week to place something called an "IVC filter," which is designed to stop blood clots from breaking loose and traveling to dangerous places in the body like the lungs, heart, or brain. Having the IVC filter will not stop blood clots from developing in the first place (I will likely still develop them from time to time), but the filter should keep them from becoming deadly.

I came off the blood thinner last week. The blood loss is notably less than before, which should improve my red blood counts and energy level.

I am writing this chapter from my airplane seat on a flight to Houston to begin a week of scans and procedures at MD Anderson. This trip is being done in anticipation of entering a Phase 1 immunotherapy clinical trial. I have eleven events scheduled over four days. If nothing disqualifying turns up on these CT scans, MRIs, blood draws, etc., I will return next week to finalize the process of being accepted into the clinical trial, which will be a fairly invasive and time-consuming process over the next several months.

Entering a Phase I clinical trial is daunting and not for the faint of heart. The decision process is made somewhat easier when you are running out of FDA-approved treatment options and your cancer continues to progress. That is the crossroads where I now find myself. A Phase I clinical trial has - as its main purpose - determining the maximum safe amount of drug that can be given to patients before they begin to experience "serious adverse events" (you know, the stuff you hear on the TV commercials that scares the **** out of you and you wonder "why would anyone in their right mind take that drug?")

A Phase I trial is a "first in man" trial, meaning it is the first time that the drug, or drug combination, has been given to humans. I have had more than one oncologist tell me that, sadly, Phase I clinical trials are not for the benefit of patients, but rather for the pharmaceutical companies conducting the trial. But even still, there is some amount of efficacy data that can be gleaned from the trial and hopefully, as the dosage increases, some therapeutic benefit will result.

Many years ago, I proudly represented a CRO (contract research organization) that does clinical research on behalf of pharmaceutical companies. I was the Global Controller and I vividly remember my first quarter, brand-new in the chair, where we met as a finance team to discuss projected financial results for the current quarter prior to meeting with our investors.

Although I was proud to be involved with a company that does clinical research, I knew absolutely nothing about the business of clinical trials. I think everyone can relate to being in a setting where you are completely ignorant of the topic(s) being discussed, yet also feeling the need to say something intelligent and look somewhat relevant to the process.

Our Chief Financial Officer — who also happens to be a long-time, dear friend of mine — was laying the groundwork for disappointing quarterly financial results because one of the clinical trials for which there appeared to be great promise (and ultimately, significant revenue) — had to be canceled. When questioned by our CEO about what was going on with that trial, our CFO said, "the monkey died."

As a lifelong, unabashed animal lover, I was immediately saddened by hearing that a monkey died but quite frankly, I had no idea what the **** he was talking about. There was a palpable sense of disappointment in the room that was no doubt a mixture of sadness for the monkey, but also for the financial repercussions of the trial being canceled. I held on for dear life for the rest of the meeting, desperately hoping that I did not have to make some sort of intelligent comment about the trial's cancellation.

After the meeting, I went directly to our CFO and asked what "the monkey died" meant. It was then that I learned that clinical trials have a preclinical phase, where a drug or drug combination is trialed in animals (often mice) before it ever gets tested on a human being. Once safety is established in a preclinical model, it can then go into a human for the first time, in a Phase I clinical trial.

If accepted into the trail at MD Anderson, I will be receiving a trial drug combination that has never been tested on a human being before (note: I later learned that I was the only person in the world in this trial). I know from reading the "informed consent" that a few patients (nearly 10%, in fact) in the initial dosing succumbed to the clinical trial itself, requiring a reformulation of the drug combination. This is the current challenge and the promise of immunotherapy. It offers such great promise for the future by figuring out how to re-arm the body's own immune system to eradicate cancer cells, yet do it in a way that keeps the immune system from going into full-blown, seek-and-destroy mode. This state, known as "cytokine release syndrome," results when the immune system gets so charged up that it also begins destroying things other than the target, including otherwise healthy tissue and organ function. This can be a lethal reaction.

If I qualify for the trial, I will have to sign documents acknowledging this risk. I don't take it lightly. The daughter of a dear friend of mine — Sophia Kappen — died at the tender age of six years old while fighting leukemia in a CAR-T clinical trial. Her parents did everything imaginable to fight her cancer, all to a crushing, disappointing result.

A friend of mine from Cincinnati Bell — Will Kays — died while participating in a clinical trial at MD Anderson a few years ago. Will was the image of the high school quarterback - handsome and fit. He had it all. Will's case was particularly unfortunate — he was a nonsmoker that took great care of himself and was diagnosed with advanced lung cancer. He came to see us at Cincinnati

Cancer Advisors while he was going back-and-forth to MD Anderson. His visit to CCA rekindled our friendship from many years ago working together at Cincinnati Bell. We were going to have lunch together after his next visit to MD Anderson. We exchanged updated contact information and talked general timelines to get together. We never had that lunch because he died shortly thereafter... shortly after participating in Ride Cincinnati, once again the picture of health, all while battling a deadly disease.

These next several months will be tough. I will try to find the humor in it all. When I see it, you will hear about it. I will spend longer apart from my wife, family, and my dogs than I have ever had to before. I am sad just thinking about it, but you fight the fight in front of you when you have cancer.

This is about the closest thing to a high-stakes bet that this risk-averse, recovering accountant will ever make. I am having to move fast... updating the last will and testament and medical directives, getting a more complicated than normal tax return filed, getting the house refinanced, explaining to Diana the ins and outs of paying the family bills, etc.

We take for granted what goes into drug development and how many drugs on the market allow us to live a near normal life, despite otherwise debilitating or life-threatening conditions. As much as I hate the thought of it, sometimes animals die and sometimes people with families die all in pursuit of therapies that will allow us to live better, longer lives.

My guess is that almost everyone participating in a cancer-based clinical trial is there due to some measure of desperation, but they are nonetheless people that we owe a great debt of gratitude to prior clinical trial participants for helping to get us where we are today.

Based on all these developments, our 40th anniversary trip to France and Monaco now looks like a pipe dream, but I still look forward to returning to a life where cancer is not pummeling my body. I think of Rocky III, where Clubber Lang (Mr. T) is kicking the living **** out of Rocky Balboa, but the fight is not over yet. Rocky is taking the punches repeatedly in the "rope-a-dope" fashion that I mentioned in a prior chapter. Even when it looks hopeless, you know that Rocky can still rally...and will rally. I am by no means Rocky Balboa in this scenario, but I do know from experience that the human body can take a lot of punishment and somehow still manage to go on. I am betting on that.

[Postscript: as I mentioned above, I wrote this chapter while on the flight to Houston. Before the plane landed, I received a text message from the Clinical Trial Coordinator at MD Anderson that said "Please call as soon as possible. It's about the financial clearance for your participation in the trial". The first thing I thought to myself — of course — was "Houston, we have a problem" and indeed we did. Now it was a matter of waiting to see whether my insurance company would do the right thing by listening to some of the top genitourinary cancer specialists in the world, so they will understand why the recommended course of treatment is necessary, and ultimately approve it. If they don't, the time, effort and money spent getting here will have all been a waste, and I don't know what my remaining options are.]

STAYIN' ALIVE

BIG day today. My calendar was jammed with a multitude of different appointments scheduled for everything from simple blood work, urinalysis, bone scan, FDG PET scan, and a brain MRI at, of all times, 10:15 p.m.

As I tromp around the concrete jungle that is the MD Anderson (dozens of health systems comprising the largest employer within the state of Texas) wearing shorts, t-shirt, sneakers, exhibiting my hairless chicken legs and bony, flat-as-a-pancake rear end, mesh sleeve covering my dangling IV catheter, and of course, with trusty leather briefcase in hand, I am quite the picture of cool. For some inexplicable reason, the image of John Travolta strutting down a street in "Saturday Night Fever" popped into my head and gave me a good laugh.

Whether you like Barry Gibb's falsetto or not (personally, it makes me want to want to tear my eardrums out), the song is iconic and still as catchy as ever. Even a non-dancer, after consuming a plentiful amount of liquid courage, might be tempted to get up and make a fool of yourself upon hearing this song. It's not a layup like doing the "Electric Slide" at a wedding, but I don't know how anyone stays seated when "Stayin' Alive" is playing at high volume.

It's the lyrics that made me laugh when I thought about it this morning, especially, *"Well, you can tell by the way I use my walk, I'm a woman's man, no time to talk."*

Thanks to the cancer-related compression fractures in my spine, I don't really "walk" these days. It's more like a determined hobble, accompanied by a pronounced grimace. I am hoping against hope that I will get some relief next week in the form of a "kyphoplasty," a procedure where a special type of medical grade "cement" will be injected into my vertebrae. The goal is to restore the vertebrae's height and rebuild it, while also relieving the associated pain.

I'm a woman's man, eh? Hardly. First, I am fortunate enough to have the only woman I would ever want or will ever need. Secondly, thanks to nine years of hormone therapy, my male equipment no longer works for anything other than the most basic of needs. In fact, after nine years of testosterone deprivation, I am pretty much a woman in a man's body, so I wouldn't even know what to do with a woman even if I caught one these days.

"Feel the city breakin' and everybody shakin'..."

The only people shaking these days when they see me coming are the claims processors for my insurance company who have been billed $330,841.19 (and for which they have already been paid $97,686.81) since the beginning of 2024, a mere 105 days ago as I write this. By the time I am done with a weeks' worth of scans and procedures here at MD Anderson, I suspect that the top number will be well over $400,000, or roughly $4,000 a day in billed claims since the beginning of the year.

I have touched on the treatment toxicity and financial toxicity that comes with having cancer. I am so fortunate that we have good health insurance and have rarely had a claim or request for pre-authorization denied (stay tuned on that though — there are some ominous developments on that front with respect to my next batch of treatments). The thing is... I have no doubt that the number of claims that have been submitted to my insurance coverage would be a lot higher than if I wasn't invested in my own care, or easily took no for an answer.

Metastatic cancer requires constant vigilance and an aggressive approach to treatment. I think of it in terms of doing everything I can possibly do to keep punching it in the head so it can't move forward. And yet, even with that aggressive approach, the last six months have proven that cancer will eventually find a way to break through. I worry about patients that are not able to advocate for themselves, or do not have a person or organization that can help them do that.

"You know it's alright, it's okay, I'll live to see another day."

That's really what this current visit is all about. Over the last decade, I have pretty much cycled through all forms of FDA-approved treatment for advanced prostate cancer with moderate success. There's not really anything left from an FDA-approved standpoint at this time. The most recent "next big thing" in advanced prostate cancer treatment — PSMA-targeting treatments such as Pluvicto — yielded phenomenal results for me for a limited amount of time but once again... cancer figured out a new pathway, so it's unlikely that I will be able to go on Pluvicto again.

I've already done chemotherapy with limited success, but I am now resistant to hormone therapy and my body is pretty much a shooting gallery for targeted radiation. But I must be careful with radiation these days as it is now causing treatment-related complications and continued radiation that has a depressing effect on lymphocyte production, which could potentially limit the effectiveness of immunotherapy in the future.

But it's alright, it's okay, because there is always the next glimmer of hope and for me, it's immunotherapy. Until very recently, immunotherapy against prostate cancer was pretty much a dismal failure that offered little hope to advanced prostate cancer patients, but things are changing rapidly. The clinical trial that I hope to be entering is for what's known as a "bispecific antibody conjugate" treatment. Simply put, bispecific antibodies work by connecting a cancer cell to an immune system cell, disrupting cancer's signaling pathways and allowing the immune system's T cells to destroy the cancer cells. I suspect (but won't know for sure until I talk to my medical oncologist) that the game changer is once again the PSMA PET scan technology that allows the T-cell to be trained to recognize the prostate cancer cell, latch onto it, and destroy it.

The hope is that I will pass the thirteen screenings I have here in Houston this week, therefore able to enter the clinical trial, and that I can persuade my insurance company to approve the three-week hospital stay that will be required during the first few infusions. If all of that happens, and I tolerate the dosage without any serious adverse effects (which would get me kicked out of the trial), I do believe — much to my insurance company's chagrin — I will be stayin' alive for a good deal longer. But trust me, all the ladies are safe.

CLINICAL TRIAL, OR CRIMINAL TRIAL?

EVER since I arrived in Houston for the pre-trial testing, pretty much every functioning part of my body (as well as a few non-functioning parts) has been scoped, probed, poked, prodded and in some cases, twisted - as part of thirteen separate procedures to establish my "baseline" before entering the clinical trial.

I can honestly say that I have never felt so exhausted in my entire life. I have spent these last two weeks running to appointments and procedures (sometimes three a day) across the massive MD Anderson medical campus. I told the clinical trial coordinator yesterday that I have both test fatigue and test result fatigue.

Every single test result is a nail biter, as it is up to the clinical trial sponsor to decide what the tolerance level is for any test result that strays from "normal." Yesterday was spent doing two "re-tests" because there were a few things in the original tests that the trial sponsor wasn't happy with. Even on the re-test, there were still some concerns, but the deviations were largely explainable by recent events. So the trial sponsor is ok with proceeding, which means I have been accepted into the clinical trial (but wait, as always, there is more to the story).

That means I will check into a hospital room here at MD Anderson tomorrow afternoon to get settled. Then we begin blood collection, vital signs, etc. in anticipation of starting the first infusion the following morning. I did receive a pleasant surprise in going over the hospitalization schedule with the clinical trial coordinator yesterday. I was under the impression that once I checked into the hospital, I would be hospitalized until I was cleared following the third infusion, which would be three weeks from now. As it turns out, if I tolerate the treatments well and don't exhibit any signs or symptoms of "cytokine release syndrome," I can be hospitalized each Sunday and be checked out of the hospital each Wednesday, allowing me to leave the hospital environment for the other half of the week. That has its own obvious benefits, and it also allayed the concerns I had about the ability to keep up with my job in the meantime, from the friendly confines of a hospital room.

Back to this clinical trial acceptance process. It has been amusing, enraging, exhausting and at times, has felt a bit like being cross-examined by a district attorney. I did not have a full appreciation of how medical records follow you around through life until I went through this clinical trial acceptance process.

During the prelude to clinical trial acceptance, I had already spent many hours on the phone going through my medical history. Like LOTS of hours. Nonetheless, only days before the scheduled pretrial hospital admittance date, I received a phone call from my slightly breathless clinical trial coordinator at

8:30 p.m. She said she needed to clarify a few things on my medical record before sending my information to the clinical trial sponsor. There was a palpable sense of urgency to the call, given the tight timeline for acceptance and the beginning of the trial. I was frustrated that we had to spend even more time on this, but I knew that I wasn't the one holding the cards, so I rolled my eyes, sighed a bit, sucked it up, and said "Ok, what do you need to know?"

This call went on for at least another ninety minutes and I was amazed by the questions.

One of my favorite exchanges went something very close to this ("CTC" refers to my clinical trial coordinator):

CTC: "So, how long have you had asthma?"

Me: "I'm not sure how to answer because I don't have asthma."

CTC: "But it says here that you have asthma."

Me: "Again, I'm not sure what to tell you but I can tell you that I don't have asthma."

CTC: "So, do you have any idea why your medical record says that?"

Me (after thinking about it for a minute): "The only thing I can think of is that when I was a very young man — at least 30 years ago - I would get annual bronchial infections. My family doctor eventually referred me to an allergist to try to figure out why."

CTC: "So, did he tell you had asthma?"

Me: "No, but he did test me for allergies, put me on allergy shots for many years, and documented that I had 'chronic allergic rhinitis'."

CTC: "What is chronic allergic rhinitis?"

Me (now getting frustrated): "Whether most people that live in the Ohio River Valley know it or not, they likely have chronic allergic rhinitis. It's basically "allergies" - runny nose, watery eyes, coughing, sneezing, and feeling like you have a cold all spring and summer long."

CTC: "What do you do to manage that?"

Me: "I take a 10 mg tablet of Claritin each day."

CTC: "So, you don't have asthma then?"

Me: "Nope."

CTC: "OK, I'll explain this to the trial sponsor, but they may have more questions because your medical record says that you have asthma."

Me: "I'm not really sure what else to say at this point."

This same type of back-and-forth went on over a documentation that I have "irritable bowel syndrome," which I also don't have, all due to a visit to a gastroenterologist more than 30 years ago, with no findings (so "irritable bowel syndrome" became the default diagnosis).

This also continued with discussions of the documented "traumatic brain injury" from a skiing accident in early 2000 that turned out to be a concussion and an eye socket fracture, with no long-term negative effects nor any structural brain issues noted or detected.

I was also asked about when my doctor first told me that I had "metastatic castrate-resistant prostate cancer." I said that despite knowing that is how my cancer is classified, none of my doctors — and I have many — have ever said to me that I have "metastatic castrate-resistant prostate cancer." She said, "this makes things tricky, since we really need to establish that on the timeline." I said — "once again, I'm not sure what to tell you."

Getting into a clinical trial, and particularly a brand-new clinical trial, is not for the faint of heart, but there may come a time in your life when it is required or represents your best shot at spending additional time here on Earth. Based on my experience, it requires the right combination of compliance, diligence, patience, humility, and more patience, all of which needs to be supplemented with a heavy dose of sheer determination.

I wonder how many other people there are out there who don't realize the implication of some of these stray items that become part of their permanent medical record. After 90 minutes of frustration working through these "clarifications" the other evening, the same diagnoses still appeared in my chart two days later when I met with my nurse practitioner, when we had to go through them all again. Seriously?

This all becomes particularly problematic when your disease journey causes you to move in and out of multiple medical systems, where you must supply the same information, and try to correct misinformation in your medical record, over-and-over-again. Despite the billions of dollars that have been spent by hundreds of health systems across the country on the vaunted Epic electronic medical records system, it does not integrate that information nearly as well as a patient might hope, especially when the chips are down and quick action is required.

Each year, Diana and I receive a report from the Social Security Administration showing what our monthly social security benefit would be if we were to take retirement at various points in time. This report also lists the maximum amount of wages each year that this calculation is based on. Despite moving our residence multiple times, getting married, and changing jobs a countless number of times, I have never found an error in this report. It's fascinating to me that this information is driven off one number, issued to you at/near birth, that follows you around through life. This social security numbering system was developed by the oft-criticized U.S. government, with the first social security numbers issued to people in 1936.

After going through all of this, it occurs to me that there is not an equivalent "medical records number" when it comes to your health… a single number issued at/near birth that allows your medical information to follow you through life. That way, patients would not be expected to scramble to answer these types of questions when time may be of the essence and - not to over dramatize - but when their life might be on the line. I am not naïve — I know it may not be seamless, especially if one medical professional does not agree with the conclusion of another, but there must be a way to do this for the purposes of a workable medical record that is consistent across medical systems.

Perhaps there are practical considerations beyond my level of comprehension, but I would submit that most any argument against the ability to do something like this would have been met with a similar argument back when the U.S. government was contemplating issuing social security numbers for the first time. Somehow, saddled by bureaucracy, and using comparatively primitive computing technology (i.e., virtually none), the U.S. government managed to pull it off. Now, ironically enough, your social security number has since become an integral part of your medical record. It feels like we as a country should do a better job at this.

STEVE ABBOTT

FAILURE TO LAUNCH

*THIS chapter is devoted to the many good souls that donate their pint of blood —
not for money, glory, the chocolate chip cookies, or any "swag" they may get by do-
nating blood, but because they believe it's the right thing to do. Ironically, prior to
the beginning of my cancer journey, I would have probably been considered a bor-
derline "trypanophic," with a propensity to avoid needle sticks whenever possible.
As such, I never donated blood and by the time I knew the value of doing so and
wanted to do it, I was ineligible due to the radiation I had already undergone, and
the chemotherapy I would eventually undergo. I feel safe in saying that I will never
be eligible to donate blood again, so I feel about our members of the military as I do
about those that donate blood — people that put on their big boy and big girl pants
and make sacrifices for their fellow citizens, in many (most?) cases for the benefit of
people they will never meet. Cincinnati, Ohio has a renowned institution named
the Hoxworth Blood Center — an organization that works tirelessly to ensure
an adequate blood supply for all Greater Cincinnatians. We should all consider
supporting these types of organizations with our donations — both hematological
and financial — as I am living proof that you never know when you might need
the help of one of these amazing organizations.*

I generally have too much pride to either (a) re-use a chapter title without an awfully good reason, or (b) default to a cliche and overused phrase like
"Houston, we have a problem" (ugh, I just did it, it's irresistible!). Anyway, you
might already be able to figure out where this is going.

Today is my clinical trial launch day, which feels appropriate given that I
am writing this from my new home-away-from-home, Houston, Texas — a city
with an innumerable number of nicknames, not the least of which is "Space
City," as it is home to NASA's Lyndon B. Johnson Space Center — one of the
most fascinating places that you will ever step foot into.

One of my nurses woke me up at about 7 a.m. saying that there had been
a few "problems" turn up in my overnight blood work that were "of concern"
that had to be addressed by the co-Principal Investigators of the clinical trial and the clinical trial sponsors, as there are more parameters to be met or
exceeded for entry into this trial than Houston has nicknames. The biggest
problem was a sudden and unexpected drop in my hemoglobin, which had
dropped from 9.3 (already at anemia levels) to 8.1 in one day's time. The normal hemoglobin level for a 61-old male varies somewhat depending on the
source, but most credible sources would put it somewhere between 13 to 17.
However, entry into a clinical trial requires a new manner of thinking. For

the most part, it really doesn't matter what is considered normal for the purposes of a routine blood test. The main thing that now matters is the parameter set for entry into - and continued participation in the trial - that the trial sponsor has set. The sponsor of my clinical trial has set that number at 8.5, and I could only proffer a pitiful 8.1.

After checking with the sponsor, the nurse told me that they needed to collect more blood and re-test to see if perhaps the hemoglobin result from the overnight draw was somehow incorrect, especially considering the significant one-day drop. That second draw would be tested and if it came back above 8.5, we still had time to go with "pre-meds" at 9:30 a.m. and the clinical trial drug injection at 10 a.m.

About an hour later, my nurse returned and said "well, that was better, but not good enough." I asked her for the second result, and she said it was 8.3. Nonetheless, she said the MD Anderson trial team was going to check with the sponsor to see if that was "close enough." Unfortunately (or perhaps, fortunately in this case), there was no "give" in the number and a blood transfusion would be required. The hope was that my hemoglobin would get up to acceptable trial levels in a few short hours so that we could make the new 1 p.m. deadline for starting the trial.

My own blood now had to be "typed." Having your blood typed in advance of a blood transfusion is necessary since not everyone can even hazard a guess at their own blood type (it happens) or may even be under the wrong impression as to their own blood type. An hour or so later, my blood type was confirmed as O+ and the MD Anderson lab began their work to prepare the bag o' blood that I would soon be receiving, from a donor I will never meet. Within an hour, the blood to be transfused had arrived at my room. Never having had a blood transfusion before, the decision was made to be very conservative in transfusing it, going slowly so the nursing staff could monitor for any adverse reactions. As a result, the transfusion itself took much longer to administer than I initially expected, and the sands were quickly slipping through the hourglass. By 1:30 p.m., the trial had been called off for the day. We will try again tomorrow.

I know I have mentioned this before, but one of the skills that cancer patients must develop, or hone, is anxiety management. There are so many test results, some that carry high stakes and for which results are not delivered instantly. Another skill you must develop and maintain is being patient.

I think back to the advice my mother — Barbara Carol Abbott — who has been largely under celebrated to this point in the book, gave me long ago.

She told me not long after my diagnosis that "you have to live based on how you feel — not based on how you might feel someday." It has taught me much, and I have pulled strength from it more times than I can count over these last (almost) 11 years of navigating a cancer journey. In this case, I quickly remembered that today I feel pretty good, and I still believe that there is reason for hope. It reminded me to focus on the positive of what the clinical trial might ultimately deliver rather than worrying about whether these new developments were going to keep me out of the trial.

To be clear, challenges still remain, some of which could prove to be significant. I recently had a close call with kidney dialysis that was the result of past cancer treatments. I have had anemia for some time now, and the problem is getting worse. Is there internal bleeding that is being caused by something else, perhaps a whole new problem altogether? We will have to get to the bottom of that soon. My cancer-related back pain is still out there — it disrupts my life in all new ways, each and every day. For the first time, my liver enzymes were all out of whack — and I mean WAY out of whack — this morning. Why? Is there something new going on that could even be a complication of past treatment or is it something current and acute? Will the same set of numbers to be there tomorrow morning?

There is a good deal to worry about if I choose to go that route, but I know that the most important thing right now is cancer control. The hope is that this new form of systemic treatment — immunotherapy — may begin to assert some lasting control over my cancer. Some members of the MD Anderson staff have been in my room telling me that once we start the trial, that I need to "visualize" my body's own killer T cells switching back on, latching on to the cancer cells, and killing them. It has been a surprising view coming from trained medical professionals, but my guess is that, by now, they have been able to correlate some outcomes with the mental approach and coping mechanisms that some patients have carried into the trials. What possible harm can come from visualizing a positive outcome? Is the idea of a killer immune cell latching on to a rogue cancer cell and killing it that far-fetched? If you think about it, that gobbling-up approach worked almost every time for Pac Man, that beloved video game icon of the 1980's.

Yes, Scarlett, tomorrow is another day. Priority #1 is getting the trial started and then doing everything that I can do from this hospital bed to maintain eligibility for the trial and optimize my own results. I will do my part, and I will trust an immunotherapy clinical trial and one of the world's most respected cancer treatment centers to do their part. I am lucky to be here, but I just want to kick this thing, get home, and see my family, friends, co-workers, and dogs, and enjoy every day I have with them.

EPILOGUE #1

AN epilogue provides the writer an opportunity to offer additional thoughts and tie up a few loose ends. My original premise was to write a simple, light-hearted blog with each entry clocking in at 500 words. The idea was that I could occasionally update my family and friends on my progress over a multi-year cancer journey, with a goal of keeping it breezy and informative, based on my own learnings (a secondary goal of this fledgling marketing guy was to build additional content in our Cincinnati Cancer Advisors website, which might increase our SEO rankings).

As someone with no medical training, it requires constant discipline to not act like I know more than I actually know about my evolving cancer journey. My desire to be a well-informed and educated patient — even to the point of working daily with some of the most intelligent medical professionals I have ever met — has still left me woefully unprepared to explain the inner workings of cancer or give seemingly well-informed advice to other patients.

As such, I have tried to fervently avoid doing that during my now 11-year battle with metastatic, castrate-resistant prostate cancer.

While there have been more than a few dark days, I would still say there are more "high-five" days. To be clear, cancer has taken a lot of things away from me, but there are so many things that cancer can never touch. As N.C. State's basketball coach Jim Valvano once said in one of the greatest speeches of all time — at the 1993 Espy Awards — in describing the physical abilities that cancer had taken away from him but citing the things that cancer could NOT rob him of, "It cannot touch my mind. It cannot touch my heart. And it cannot touch my soul."

It's cruelly ironic that Coach Valvano maintained that view despite what cancer had already done to his brain. He had to be literally helped to and from the stage by Dick Vitale (now also a cancer philanthropist and cancer survivor himself) and Coach Mike Krzyzewski, who is also a cancer philanthropist who has done amazing work for the V Foundation. It had affected his brain to the degree that he couldn't walk normally anymore. But it had not touched his mind, which is obvious when you watch the speech (if you haven't seen the speech, please run — don't walk — to watch it).

Strangely, I would submit that cancer has touched my mind, heart, and soul, but all in a good way. Perhaps it's a matter of perspective. Coach Valvano had become a very celebrated and successful college basketball coach, winning the men's national championship in 1983 with a group of kids who were never given a snowball's chance in hell at being able to pull off that miracle. That national championship final is still widely regarded as one of the greatest college basketball games in history. He had become a beloved and iconic personality in nearly every respect.

Given the amount of money that the college game now generates, the lucrative, long-term contracts that college basketball coaches can claim these days, and the television analyst gigs they are offered at the sunset of their coaching careers, it could be argued that cancer was robbing Coach Valvano of all of that, so perhaps his way to cope was to focus on what cancer could NOT take from him.

At the time of my diagnosis, I was a fun-loving and (I hope) affable guy who was muddling his way through life alongside great friends, doing work that I was not passionate about and, to be quite honest, pretty much taking each day for granted. Without some sort of shake-up, I may have just continued mailing it in, playing out the string, or whatever other metaphor you might want to use it to describe a guy that could have, and should have, done more with his life.

Cancer changed all of that for me. Whereas it could be argued that cancer robbed Coach Valvano of his future, it gave me a the chance to get out of my comfort zone, treat each-and-every day as a gift, stop wasting time doing things that I didn't want to do, and begin finding ways to — as my dear friend Janine Sharell would say - use my superpowers for good.

Common sense would tell you that any cancer patient would like to erase that diagnosis from their mind and if given the choice, make it such that it never happened. My answer might surprise you. Barring some sort of Earth-shaking medical miracle, cancer is going to shorten my lifespan. I know that. That means less years to do things with, but I feel like with getting the age-50-kick-in-the-pants that I received, I might actually eke out more "living years' than I might have otherwise.

Will I miss being with Diana, my family, friends, co-workers, and dogs if "the end" comes much earlier than I would have chosen? Of course, but that would be the case whether I lived to be 65 or 85 years of age. Thanks to recent diagnosis and treatment advances, I have already lived longer than expected, but I have no intention of giving up any time soon. I have found my voice and my purpose, and I intend to use it like a battering ram against cancer for as long as I possibly can.

Diana and I canceled our dream 40th anniversary trip when I was given the opportunity to pursue a novel therapy that could yield life-extending benefits for me. I need to be here, doing my own part to improve my outcome by extending my own life. The downside is maybe never seeing Paris and Monte Carlo, but the upside could be adding more years to my life and having more time this summer to sit on my back patio and enjoy the company of Diana and the dogs.

I am pleased to report that I did receive the first dose of the trial medicine today. I am being monitored very, very closely by the medical team here at MD Anderson and everything is fine as I close out the first day after treatment. Now I need to do everything in my power to hang on to this clinical trial like Harrison Ford hung onto the Nazi truck's muffler in "Raiders of the Lost Ark" or Robert DeNiro did in "Cape Fear" (a great, albeit highly unbelievable movie scene, but who cares?).

I have taken up a good deal of your time sharing my cancer journey. I hope it has been helpful in some way. It has caused me to rediscover my lost passion for writing, and I hope, use my superpowers for good. Perhaps you have this book because it somehow caught your eye at an independent bookstore somewhere. Maybe you are a cancer survivor. Maybe you are battling cancer now or supporting a family member or friend with cancer. Perhaps you donated to one of my favorite charities — Cincinnati Cancer Foundation, Inc. (federal employer ID number 81-4093626) or you are a patient of Cincinnati Cancer Advisors, and you received a free copy as part of your consultation. No matter how you may have received the book, I am humbled that you accepted it and that you are reading it. I intend to continue publishing updates online, and those updates will hopefully be added to a future edition of the book.

My hope is that those future updates will find me triumphing over cancer for many more years to come. For as long as I can continue proudly representing the Cincinnati Cancer Foundation, you can find the updates at www.cincinnaticanceradvisors.org/abbottjourney.

I have titled this chapter "Epilogue 1" because I anticipate several more epilogues as my fight against cancer continues. By doing it as a charity fundraising project for Cincinnati Cancer Advisors, I hope that many cancer patients will benefit either directly or indirectly from this book for several years to come. Thank you for being a crucial part of my cancer journey, as well as my life's journey.

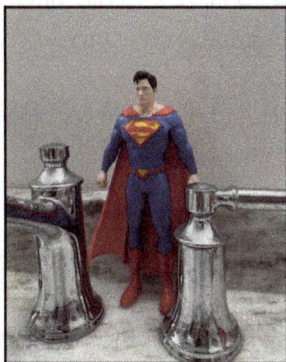

SUPERMAN

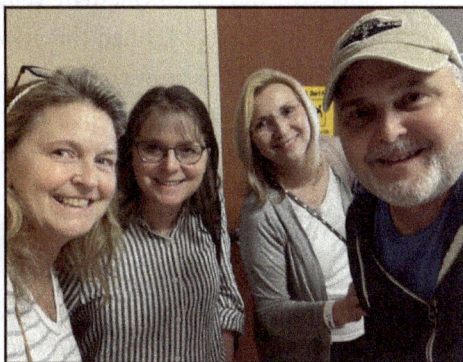

Left: *Miniature Superman statue given to me by my sister, Debbie McNeil. It sits atop my bathroom counter as a daily reminder to keep up the fight against advanced prostate cancer. Right: My sisters (left to right) Lisa Moore and Debbie McNeil during their multi-day visit with Diana and myself at MD Anderson Cancer Center at Houston, Texas.*

THIS chapter is dedicated to my sisters, Debbie McNeil and Lisa Moore. They recently "walked the cancer walk" with me by coming to Houston as I started my clinical trial at MD Anderson. Debbie brought with her an assortment of Superman related items...a blanket, two pairs of Superman dress socks, a Superman-themed poem that she wrote on my behalf, and even a little Superman statue that now adorns my bathroom sink as a reminder of her kindness. The next few chapters will call her generous assessment of me as Superman into open question and remind us all that Superman had his own issue to deal with... called Kryptonite.

It has been almost two months since I last wrote upon entry into the clinical trial. I have missed it. To be clear, if there is one thing these last seven weeks have taught me — at least from a physical point of view — is that I am no Superman.

My first trial drug medication at MD Anderson was administered on April 29, 2024. Following that first dose, I was cautious but brimming with confidence and hope. For two solid weeks of hopscotching across the sprawling MD Anderson campus, in and out of rideshare vehicles to make it to the (often invasive) next scan, test or biopsy, I had the prize in mind...acceptance into the clinical trial that had been recommended to me.

I had run all the tricks and traps I needed to get into the trial but strangely, there were a few things I didn't know at the time I entered the trial:

1. This was a Phase I, "first in man" trial, meaning it was the first time this drug, at this strength, had ever been given to a human being.
2. Not only was it a first-in-man trial, but as noted previously, I was also the only person in the world that was in the trial. Nobody else, just this so-called Superman.
3. The first dose I received was the "baby" dose, followed by the "transition" dose at 10 times the strength of the baby dose. The third dose — the "target" dose would be 10 times the strength of the transition dose, or more than 100 times the strength of the baby dose. Uh... what?

None of these three facts were withheld from me. I certainly understood #1, especially having worked for a contract research organization in the past. Uncharacteristically for me, I just had not asked the questions that would have led me to #2 or #3. Little did Superman know, but he was about three weeks to the day from getting his a** royally kicked.

The baby dose was a bit of a yawner... some inflammation at the injection site and a brief flirtation with a fever as the trial drug medicine began drawing the curious attention of my immune system. The level of monitoring from the clinical trial team certainly seemed disproportionate relative to the amount of reaction my body gave to the trial drug. Thankfully, my wife Diana was there to keep me company, because most of the time was spent laying in a hospital bed, counting the minutes until I could get discharged, roughly 72 hours from the time of each injection.

The inpatient component of this trial — whereby I had to check into the hospital and stay there for three days at a time for monitoring — was not terrible at first, but it was completely incompatible with my still go -go-go lifestyle at 61 years of age. Even though I felt fine after injection #1, it was nonetheless very difficult to be largely isolated from almost everything I care about... my family, dogs, friends and even my job. And I have to do this twice more after this?

In hindsight, I now look back on injection #1 as the "good ol' days" of my clinical trial experience.

THERE'S NO PLACE LIKE HOME (ESPECIALLY WHEN YOU CAN'T GET THERE)

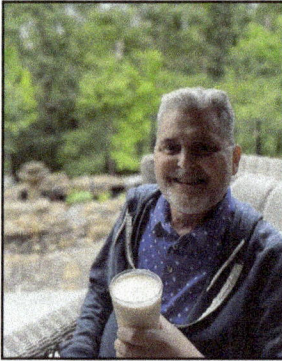

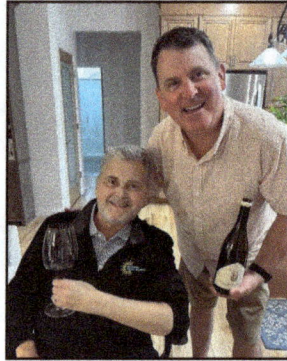

Left: Despite our best intentions to enjoy our 40th wedding anniversary overseas, I was more than happy to enjoy my back patio, milkshake in hand, overlooking the new water feature Diana installed as an anniversary gift. There's no place like home. Right: Steve enjoying a visit from his brother, Brad Abbott.

ONE thing that I neglected to mention in the last chapter was that trial drug injection #1 was not without incident, despite being administered at the premier cancer treatment facility in the United States. There was something that I would come to learn quickly, which is that the trial drug had to be formulated onsite by the "investigational pharmacy" because... well... it's the only place that drug is being given and the short "half-life" in getting it into the patient. Said another way, there is not enough time to formulate it offsite and get it into the patient before the effectiveness wanes and the drug becomes worthless.

Even though injection #1 was the "baby" dose and my immune system's response to it was largely uneventful, the pharmacy was not able to get it to me in time on that first injection day, which meant a day wasted laying in a hospital waiting for something... anything... to happen. It also pushed out my timeline as far as when I was going to be able to check out of the hospital following the 72 hours of required observation. The goal posts moved on me by one day, and in the wrong direction. In hindsight, this was an ominous development that would come to characterize the entire clinical trial experience.

What this all meant was that I would not be discharged on that first Thursday and would now barely be discharged in time to make a Friday morning consultation with my new doctor, who is also the Principal Investigator for the clinical trial. This had to be arranged for less than one hour after discharge. Exhausting. What is ultimately meant is that we did not have time to get back home for the weekend. This was the first of many disappointments in that regard.

Thankfully, MD Anderson does have a very nice hotel onsite that is run by Marriott and is perfectly situated for accessing both sides of what I would call the treatment "campus" there. That eased the burden (and unexpected expense, accompanied by unwinding all our travel arrangements home) but nonetheless, a nice hotel on the campus of a cancer treatment facility is not home.

There were other things I would come to learn during injection #2. First, if you are honest about anything that happens to your body while on the trial drug, you get a free scan of some sort! Stomach bothering you a bit? Enjoy a complimentary abdominal CT scan, courtesy of the trial sponsor! Report a minor headache and you might find yourself on the way to a brain MRI. OK, I get it... but they still gotta rule out that is the trial drug causing it.

Second (and this happened), no over-the-counter drugs without permission from the trial sponsor. A simple but persistent case of heartburn one evening left me waiting four hours to receive a Maalox tablet. Don't even get me started about the fact that I haven't been able to have a glass of wine or anything interesting to drink for almost a month now. Those that know me know that a daily glass (or two) of Napa Valley Cabernet is part of my prescription for a happy life.

All said, though, at this point, I'm still very grateful to be in a clinical trial, to still "have a shot," and not be too much worse for wear than not being able to get back to my own bed and my little posse of dogs for the weekend. But treatment #3 awaits...

THIRD TIME... NOT THE CHARM (NOTHING CHARMING ABOUT IT, IN FACT)

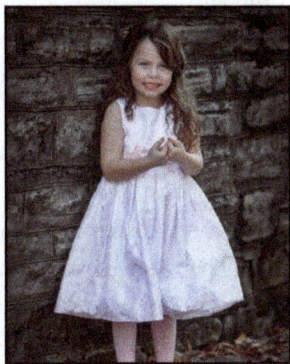

Our dear friend Amy Kappen is a tireless advocate for bereaved families following the loss of her daughter Sophia (pictured) at age 6. In addition to her work as the founder of the Best Day Ever Foundation, Amy was also honored as the Leukemia & Lymphoma Society's (LLS) "Woman of the Year" in 2018, when she raised $230,000 for LLS in ten weeks' time.

THIS chapter is dedicated to Sophia Kappen, the daughter of one of my dear friends who lost her battle with leukemia at the tender age of six years old. Sophia had an initial very encouraging response to chimeric antigen receptor T-cell therapy ("CAR-T") before her immune system went into seek-and-destroy mode. She was a victim of "cytokine release syndrome," and her loss was a stunning turn of events that is still felt deeply and will always be felt deeply by her many friends and family. Despite this tragic outcome, a new bereavement charity called the "Best Day Ever Foundation" was founded by her mother and my dear friend, Amy Kappen. Please consider supporting bereaved families at https://www.bestdayeverfoundation.us/

This now brings us to trial drug injection #3... the first injection at the "target" dose level and in this case, the highest dose of this drug that has been given to any person ever. Although the most serious effect of injection #2 appeared to be some wonky blood results with my kidneys and liver, the only real practical effect (other than the previously mentioned disappointment of not being able to get home for the weekend) was an unexpected trip to the Ambulatory Treatment Center for a "bolus" of IV fluids to help offset some dehydration that had crept in.

At the same time as I was given the fluids, I also received my (now overdue) Lupron injection. Lupron, like Eligard, is a first-line hormone therapy treatment against prostate cancer that almost all guys with prostate cancer are on for the rest of their lives, even after they become what is referred to as "castrate-resistant" or "hormone insensitive." This is because it is the best way to totally shut down the production of testosterone in the male body (mine is now regularly less than 3 nanograms per deciliter versus a "normal" of 300-1,000 nanograms per deciliter). And as a bonus, you can get the injection directly into your choice of buttocks. Whoa, good times!

The good news is that injection #3 was administered pretty much on time — perhaps no more than a one-hour delay than the anticipated time of 10 a.m. There always seemed to be some internal drama about when "pharmacy" was going to have the drug done and delivered, but today's was a minor delay at best. Since the first two injections were delivered to the stomach and injection site irritation remained, the decision was made to deliver the now two-syringe payload into my left quadricep. There was much curiosity from the nursing staff as many of them had just been selected to join the clinical trial team.

Other than just being stuck with a needle, which is as familiar to me now as getting up in the morning, it was pretty much a non-event. So much so that by 7 p.m., I told my bonus nurse (my wife Diana, who many don't know she once intended to be a nurse) that she could go get something to eat and a good night's rest. Although I was not cavalier about things and knew that the night was still young, I was able to answer the constant flow of "how are you feeling?" questions from the nursing staff and friends and family with a truthful "really good — thanks for asking.")

Everything changed starting a little after 10 p.m. Diana was back at the hotel and other than someone coming around to collect blood from me and do "vitals" every few hours, I was alone for the evening. I put a news program on the TV (I am an avowed news junkie) and tried to go off to sleep. Within an hour, I began experiencing the effects of what is known as "cytokine release syndrome." What began as bone chilling cold was, ironically, the result of a 103-degree-and-rising temperature.

My teeth were chattering and there was nothing I could do to stop it. There were no number of warm blankets that I could pile on to get warm. My nurse was notably concerned, alerting my doctor and representative of the trial drug sponsor. I try to not ever be overly dramatic with these things, but there were several hours where I honestly thought I was dying and about two of those hours when I almost wished that I did.

It was an unbelievably long night. I remember seeing a fuzzy image of the TV screen at about 4 a.m. but that is about all that I remember, other than just wanting it to be over. Thankfully, they were able to break the worst of my fever before dawn and Diana did not have to witness what I went through during that evening. All of that said, it is not lost on me that it could have been worse, and that lives have been lost along the way to CRS, all to move cancer research forward.

PARTICIPATION TROPHY

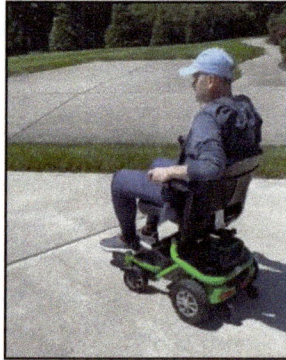

Steve trying out his new "wheels" in the driveway. This gift from friends Brian Griffin and Shelby McKee has allowed me to quickly regain my independence following spinal cord compression due to advancing prostate cancer that has metastasized to my spine.

THIS chapter is dedicated to Keith Hepp, a friend and former colleague who died tragically and unexpectedly at the age of 55 from Legionnaires Disease. As with another former Cincinnati Bell colleague of mine, Will Kays, Keith and I saw each other for the first time in years at a Leukemia & Lymphoma Society fundraiser one night where my friend Amy Kappen was being honored. We updated our mutual contact information, vowed to have lunch "sometime soon," and never did because of his untimely passing. I have lost friends way too early, and it is a large part of the reason why I give thanks for each day I am allowed to enjoy on this planet. It is also why I have a renewed focus on not "putting off" getting together with people that I care about.

I was originally going to go with the all-too-easy, somewhat uninventive chapter title of "Three Strikes and You're Out" to describe — **SPOILER ALERT** — my unceremonious dismissal from the clinical trial at MD Anderson on June 3, 2024, following a third injection at the full "target" dose level.

What is slightly ironic is that I was kicked out of the trial not because those injections were intolerable, but because it was determined that my disease was "progressing" despite the treatment. I am left to conclude that this decision was based largely — if not exclusively — on a rise in my PSA to 38 following an initial dip in that all-important number to slightly less than 20.

Although I say "all-important" above with respect to PSA as a diagnostic, this number alone is not a panacea, although it is a fairly reliable indicator of disease burden. Said another way, some men express a lot of PSA and don't necessarily have a problematic cancer (or cancer at all) and others may express little PSA and have a formidable cancer case to wrangle with (uh, that would be me.) My understanding was that one would not get kicked out of the trial solely based on PSA results but given that I had not had a CT scan or MRI of any soft tissue to that point, it must have been based solely on PSA progression. This has only been confirmed in writing in the form of a not-100%-definitive response to a text message I sent to the Principal Investigator for the trial.

So after six weeks of feeling pretty much like roadkill, I think I basically got a "participation trophy" for being in the trial. Thanks Mr. Abbott, you've been a lovely contestant! It was a temporary jolt. I had poured so much into this. So much running back and forth and somewhere north of $10,000 in expense incurred only to feel bad and have no known recommended path forward.

A slightly unexpected outcome was how isolated I felt for almost two months, even though I had Diana by my side for a good deal of it. Despite the somewhat comparatively generous size of my hospital room, there really was no room to work once you subtract out the hospital bed, nursing stations, furniture, bathroom, etc. Although I had my laptop with me, there was not a good way to use it and I began falling behind on my work and unable to help my colleagues at times. I hated that feeling.

As if I didn't already know, I love my work. I love where I work and I love who I work with. I am very lucky in that regard. Something caused me to think back to something that my former Cincinnati Bell colleague Keith Hepp said to me years ago that incensed me at the time, but lit a fire under me. At a time when we both worked in a sleepy accounting department at Cincinnati Bell, he said "you work to live; I live to work."

I thought this was a mouthful coming from a guy who admitted to having carpal tunnel syndrome from playing video games at his desk and listening to talk radio all day (I am pretty sure that Keith actually believed for a while that Bill & Hillary Clinton had Vince Foster killed thanks to Rush Limbaugh's lunatic ramblings). Ironically, Keith also ended up in health-care, becoming a well-respected executive in the health information exchange industry, helping to improve the way that patient information is shared between health systems, with a beneficial effect on patients.

Keith's comment made me mad at the time, but the truth is, it was the first time when I had to self-acknowledge that I was spending the majority of my time working in a job I was not passionate about (as I have noted before, cancer would later teach me the importance of not wasting that time anymore). Even though I went on to a series of positions doing work that I did not love, his comment caused me to double down on the work ethic taught to me by my parents. I wanted to be the hardest working guy in the room, even if I did not love what I did. That's what made that isolation in Houston feel even worse because I could not move things forward like I wanted to.

Back to the clinical trial. The good news about being booted out of the trial is that I was out of the trial. I was exhausted and needed a break from the constant litany of blood draws, vital signs, scans, and other procedures. Even though my cancer was still on the march, I had a short bit of time where I wasn't being subjected to it. Life was, and is, good on my back patio.

Physically, this trial exposed cracks in my foundation that I didn't even know existed and were not readily apparent to me even weeks or months before I began the trial. I even spent some time in the MD Anderson cardiac unit when I presented with "A-Fib" for the first time and began to become an unpredictable fall risk, who would pass out unexpectedly due to a new condition called "orthostatic hypotension," where my systolic blood pressure would drop up to 50 points when standing up. It is now a month later and I am still trying to recover from a few of these new maladies.

So, what next?

One of the blessings of being back home is that I was finally able to get a long overdue kyphoplasty, a procedure that will hopefully mitigate the excruciating pain I have been experiencing in my lumbar spine for nearly six months. That process ultimately led to the discovery that I also had three new tumors found in my thoracic spine which are causing compression on my spinal cord. This complicates things in a somewhat serious way as to what to do next to try to slow my cancer's growth, as all evidence indicates that it is moving very quickly. But... the excruciating back pain I was experiencing is better thanks to the surgery.

Thankfully, as of a month later, due to very careful management of the spinal cord compression through use of steroids, I have been able to avoid an invasive back surgery (called a "laminectomy") and I am able to get around thanks to a motorized scooter we lovingly call the "Green Machine" that I have on loan thanks to my good friend Shelby McKee.

The risk of paralysis (or even death) due to a worsening of the spinal cord issue does have to be carefully weighed in any next treatment decision. While we sort through that, at least I have my MD Anderson participation trophy and hopes of entering a new clinical trial that might prove more effective.

"H" IS FOR HOSPICE, AND HELL NO TO THAT!

THINGS have become a lot more "real" of late. As I write these words in July 2024, I am only about halfway to the goal I set for myself in February 2022 when I started the "5 Years, 500 Words at a Time" blog. My goal was to live at least five more years with metastatic castrate resistant prostate cancer.

I wasn't being cavalier in setting that goal, but I also had no experience with how things might go once cancer breaks out of your lymph nodes and makes it into your bones and soft tissue in a meaningful way. Talk about something getting your attention in a hurry!

Despite being a "regular" guy, I have the type of care and oversight for my cancer care that you might only expect a wealthy person or celebrity to have. Through my well-respected — and in many cases, renowned — colleagues at Cincinnati Cancer Advisors, I have the luxury of leveraging their connections to consult with some of the top prostate-cancer-focused oncologists in the country about my case.

This almost unfettered access to great care has no doubt added time to my life and for that I am truly grateful. My oncology team is what I often refer to as an "embarrassment of riches," yet having so many advisors - all of which are smarter than me - can sometimes lead to cases where it is tough to reconcile the advice you are receiving, especially when not everyone on your oncology team agrees on next steps.

At the behest (or at least suggestion) of my CCA colleagues, I have made a recent change to my oncology team by engaging a new local medical oncologist in Cincinnati. I say "local" because I am fortunate to consult with other "med-oncs" nationally. However, with respect to those national voices, it is your local medical oncologist who can and often does deliver your actual care. My colleague Jill Hunt calls him or her "your quarterback."

Less than a month ago, I had my first consultation with my new medical oncologist in Cincinnati. He first saw me at a time where things were not good at all from a physical point of view. There was a lot going wrong inside my body at the time and quite frankly, there still is. As a result, I am slowly coming to understand why he did what he did so early in our first meeting together. He said the "H" word... hospice.

His mention of hospice as a next step was brand new territory. I shot Diana a quick WTF? type glance and mustered up the only response I could think of, which was "uhhh, I wasn't thinking I would hear that today." A five-second-that-felt-like-five-minute period of awkward silence ensued where I did not embrace the idea, and he continued on. There were no "take backs."

Clinically, he is not wrong to at least mention it at this point, I suppose, yet it is still very difficult to hear and think about. I am a nearly 11-year advanced prostate cancer survivor and as such, I belong to several online communities where other prostate cancer guys gather to commiserate, seek advice, and in many cases, try to joke away this disease.

I have seen the progression in many cases where guys decide to stop treatment and "enjoy however much time I have left." Given how prostate cancer generally progresses, I think statements like those are better classified as euphemisms meaning "I just don't want to do this anymore."

At a second meeting with this new oncologist, he once again proposed that I either resume some form of systemic cancer treatment via a clinical trial, or consider hospice. It's clear that he wants me to understand where we are at in the process, which I do. I just can't bring myself to "give up" at this point.

So, with full knowledge that this next step is likely to really suck at times, I have decided to enter another clinical trial in hopes of (a) living long enough to bridge to whatever the next best treatment is and (b) be part of the "science" in getting there through clinical trial participation.

Assuming I am accepted into the new trial, I will start treatment in about 10 days. It will be on an outpatient basis, every three weeks, and it will be close to home at a treatment facility I am very familiar with. I will be close to family and friends, and I can be home instead of in a hospital 1,000 miles away where I don't know anybody. I am hopeful that the results will be better this time.

So for now, I'll respond with my own H word and say "hell, no" to the hospice idea in favor of Coach Jim Valvano's "Never Give Up" mantra. Sometime next week, it will take everything I have in me to not pull a Samuel L. Jackson in the first Jurassic Park movie and say to Diana, "hold onto your butts" when that first infusion under the new trial starts (I will probably still say it and Diana will likely just roll her eyes).

PREPARING TO DIE, WHILE YEARNING TO LIVE

SO here we go... the last chapter in what started as a breezy 500-word blog has now evolved into a short book (hopefully you don't think it has devolved after seeing the blah, bummer of a chapter title). You might be thinking, "wait, what happened to the laughing, joking around guy? Where did he go?" Don't worry, I'm still here... it's just I have a lot to think about these days.

First and foremost, my days have been filled with visits from family and friends. It seems whenever I am not sitting at my computer working on something, I have a visitor — or visitors — who sense something is wrong (but may not know the full extent of it) and want to stop by for a bit, maybe bring a meal, and just sit and chat for a while. I can't think of one of those visits (now numbering well into the twenties or thirties) that have not been fun and lighthearted in nature. I have laughed a lot as the old stories get replayed.

But yet, I know I still have work to do if I want to leave things behind for Diana in a way that I would want to leave them. Once the houseguests leave, it's back to a combination to trying to get my work done, as well as continuing to chip away with filling a 2 ½ inch binder full of (I hope) everything Diana will need to know to pay the bills, know where to find things, who to call to redeem the life insurance policy, etc. I am laser focused on making sure that... as they say... my "affairs are in order" so that she does not have to struggle any more than necessary if things go south.

Now... please don't think we are not laughing along the way. We both have a pretty good sense of gallows humor so it's not quite as heavy as it sounds. Take for example the music playlist for my "Celebration of Life" that I am planning. Because I am not going to have a traditional funeral, I call it my "fun-eral" playlist and it won't have "Amazing Grace" or other sad songs on it. It will have fun songs on it. Like "come prepared to dance" type fun music, which is highly ironic given that me dancing is a rarer sight than meeting up with Bigfoot himself. Anyway, I'll do the "reveal" on the playlist sometime soon with hopes she approves but I expect to make changes.

Our house was recently refinanced, the messy 2023 federal tax return is in the process of being finalized and filed, the beneficiary details on the life insurance policy has been confirmed and verified, my car title transferred so it won't have to go through probate, and all estate planning documents are completed, signed and notarized. I will probably never be done puttering around with the 2 ½ inch binder but it's in good enough shape now that I feel like I can get out and enjoy the back patio a bit, welcoming friends and family whenever my time and health allow.

I did have a "moment" a few weeks ago after Diana and I had one of our more serious conversations about it all. We both had to take some crying breaks along the way, but we were almost always able to bring things back home with a memory of a trip, or some silly antic from one of our dogs, or something else that made us give thanks for 45 wonderful years together (40 of them married). Nonetheless, I wrote the poem the next morning. It is an entirely new type of writing for me. Perhaps I will do more of it in the future. It's more than just lashing out at cancer, but rather a bit of a prayer designed to pay tribute to those that do the work to try to reduce cancer to something akin to a chronic disease. This is imperative so that cancer no longer robs families of loved ones, friendships of friends, and workplaces of workers.

These last days have been so hard, yet we are grateful for them.
We cry some and laugh a lot.
Regrets at things left undone are more than redeemed by gratitude
for what we have been able to do.
How many more lives have to be sacrificed to this monstrous disease,
this cancer?
Are 600,000 American lives each year not enough?
Healthy cells divide and morph erratically.
We can find it earlier, but we cannot stop it.
We can treat it more effectively, but it will not leave us be,
this monstrous disease — cancer.
Let us pray for those that do the work of combating this horrific disease.

STEVE ABBOTT

PUBLISHER'S NOTE

Being in the business of books for over forty years is a long time, but it's been a good, long time. This length of time makes it feel doubly momentous to be adding my first-ever Publisher's Note.

While one should never claim to have Seen It All, nonetheless, I have seen, read and edited a lot. Four decades of surfing an ever-shifting wave of manuscript pages and computer files, maneuvering around towering, tottering piers of books, and narrowly avoiding the tsunami of deadlines and missed typos renders the passing of time to be measured not in months or years, but instead by great books and authors I've been lucky to know.

This is one of those books.

Steve Abbott's *Survive and Advance* is unlike any other book I've been involved with before. First, and most fundamentally, it's an illuminating and heartfelt account of human courage battling mortality. An amazing story of an incredible person.

Some of you may have come to Steve's story via his blog "500 Words, 5 Years." Re-casting those blog posts which were written over time with a specific structure did provide Steve a template to use. The blogs became bricks in a verbal wall he erected between the medical triage and his cancer. The feedback he received from readers became the mortar that kept the wall, and his willpower, strong. Writing "500 Words, 5 Years" gave Steve something to lean on for structure and support when leaning was perhaps all he could do. This forum provided an emotional distance between physicians' clinical diagnoses and the profoundly personal responses that bubbled up inside.

The process of taking those blogs and weaving them into a narrative is akin to taking cotton from seeds to bolls to strands to fabric — look at what an amazing coat Steve has made for us, something that has kept him warm while also protecting us from the elements of nature. I'm thinking the seamstress in Donna Salyers might like this metaphor as well.

Regardless of the analogy, readers will be always grateful to Steve for sharing his struggles, amazed by his perseverance when others would have yielded to the ache and deteriorating health markers, and cheered by his humor in the midst of grim results. But he never quit — Steve always looked to **Survive and Advance.**

AUTHOR'S NOTE

If you made it this far, thank you. In reviewing the manuscript for this book prior to publication, it occurred to me that there are often "gaps" in the story-telling that can span months at a time. These gaps are largely driven by somewhat static periods in time where there may not have been much by new news, or I was just so busy with normal life I just didn't have time to write a new entry.

If you have felt confused at times by what seems to be an odd, or even bewildering treatment path, I've learned over time that the path and course of treatment is not linear and appears to change suddenly and without notice. Welcome to advanced prostate cancer. It has been a meandering, 10+ year journey through a variety of treatment choices, driven by changes in the cancer itself. Thankfully, it has largely been a matter of doing whatever it takes to stay one step ahead and keep the cancer from metastasizing to bones and soft tissue. By staying aggressive, informed, and doing whatever it takes to pursue the latest available treatments, I have been able to do that to the best of my ability. However, with working in an oncology practice, I never underestimate cancer and its own ability to shape shift and wreak havoc.

Thank you for reading this book, which I hope will prove helpful to many and serve as some sort of legacy in an otherwise humble life.

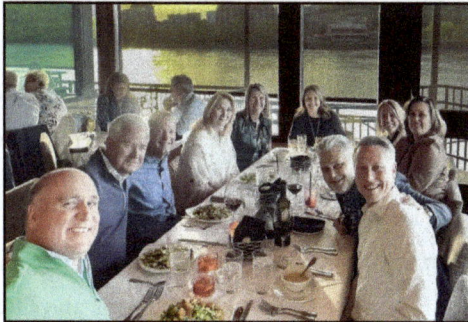

Enjoying dinner with our dearest of friends (left to right) Greg Olson, Jeff Martini, Paul McCauley, Diana Abbott, Julie McCauley, Cindy Olson, Allison Voelkerding, Katherine Martini, Steve Abbott, and Todd Voelkerding.

GLOSSARY

OF OFTEN USED TERMS (OR PEOPLE) IN THIS BOOK

The following is a layman's glossary for terms and people that you will be introduced to in this book. These are my own definitions and should not be relied on as medical information as I am not qualified to provide medical advice. I am going to describe these items in my own terms, without researching them or purporting that they are precise or are being described in a way that an oncologist would describe them.

Abbott, Diana – my wife of 40+ years and inseparable companion for more than 45 years, Diana Marie (nee Sewell) Abbott. See Chapter 45 for more on this amazing woman.

Androgen Deprivation Therapy (ADT) – ADT is generally the course of treatment prescribed for most men with prostate cancer after a first-line treatment such as a radical prostatectomy or radiation has failed to fully eradicate a man's prostate cancer. ADT works by dramatically reducing the amount of testosterone in a man's body as testosterone is believed to a source of prostate cancer growth in a man with prostate cancer.

Barrett, Dr. William L. – a prince of a man, Dr. Barrett is my long-time friend, doctor (i.e., radiation oncologist), and boss (as the founder and Chairman of the Board of the Cincinnati Cancer Foundation, Inc.).

Cincinnati Cancer Advisors (CCA) – CCA is a consultative oncology practice located in Cincinnati, Ohio that provides secondary case review, genetic counseling and testing services, and financial navigation services to more than 600 cancer patients each year, all provided free of charge to the patient and without billing to their private insurance company.

Cincinnati Cancer Foundation, Inc. (CCF) – CCF is a 501(c)(3) nonprofit organization whose mission is to reduce the suffering and mortality that often accompanies a cancer diagnosis. Although CCF is free to fund anything that falls within its mission, the vast majority of its funding is allocated to CCA.

Docetaxel / Taxotere – refers to the chemotherapy drug often administered to prostate cancer patients, generally once other forms of treatment have failed to control the cancer's spread. These terms are often used interchangeably as Taxotere is the brand name for Docetaxel.

Genitourinary – generally refers to the reproductive or urinary systems. Genitourinary cancers are what I often refer to as the "below the belt" cancers, which includes prostate cancer.

Lupron/Eligard – this injection, generally administered quarterly, is the first-line androgen deprivation therapy (ADT) treatment that most men will encounter once their oncologist has determined that they would benefit from ADT.

MD Anderson Cancer Center – located in Houston, Texas, this cancer-only treatment facility is considered by many to be the pre-eminent cancer treatment facility in the United States.

Medical Oncologist – considered by many to be the "quarterback" on one's oncology treatment team, the medical oncologist generally has training in the various methods for treating cancer such as radiation oncology, chemotherapy, hormone therapy, etc. The medical oncologist can and often does administer treatment to the patient, but their role is often limited to assessing the situation and helping determine the proper course of treatment.

Metastatic Castrate Resistant Prostate Cancer – this refers to prostate cancer that has spread beyond the local area to a distant site, or sites, and that has become resistant to ADT.

Pluvicto – this relatively new treatment in the war on advanced prostate cancer is a PSMA-targeting radioligand treatment developed by Novartis.

Principal Investigator (PI) – the Principal Investigator is the person charged with overseeing the administration of a clinical trial according to the trial sponsor's design.

Prostate Specific Antigen (PSA) – PSA is an antigen that appears on the surface of prostate cells. Although often indicative of prostate cancer at high levels, there are many conditions that can give rise to a man having PSA above undetectable levels. PSA is generally considered to be a fairly accurate measurement of disease burden in men that have been diagnosed with prostate cancer and can be determined with a simple and inexpensive blood test.

Prostate Specific Membrane Antigen (PSMA) – PSMA is a protein that is expressed on the surface of prostate cancer cells. Approximately 80% of men with prostate cancer express PSMA on the surface of their prostate cancer cells, which can allow for effective targeting through a new class of treatments called radioligand therapy.

PSMA PET Scan – This type of PET scan, approved only recently by the Food & Drug Administration, uses a specially formulated radiotracer to identify the exact location of prostate cancer cells, which can lead to the effective targeting of these cells through the use of new FDA-approved therapeutics such as Pluvicto.

www.ingramcontent.com/pod-product-compliance
Lightning Source LLC
Chambersburg PA
CBHW070829100426
42813CB00003B/544